Occupational Medicine

Multiple Chemical Sensitivity/Idiopathic Environmental Intolerance

Guest Editor:

Patricia J. Sparks, MD
Private Consultant
Occupational and Environmental Medicine
Mercer Island, Washington

STATE OF THE ART REVIEWS

Volume 15/Number 3
HANLEY & BELFUS, INC.

July–September 2000
Philadelphia

Publisher: HANLEY & BELFUS, INC.
210 South 13th Street
Philadelphia, PA 19107
(215) 546-4995
Fax (215) 790-9330
Web site: http://www.hanleyandbelfus.com

OCCUPATIONAL MEDICINE: State of the Art Reviews is included in *Index Medicus, MEDLINE, BioSciences Information Service, Current Contents* and *ISI/BIOMED, CINAHL database, and Cumulative Index to Nursing & Allied Health Literature.* Printed on acid-free paper.

OCCUPATIONAL MEDICINE: State of the Art Reviews   ISSN 0885-114X
July–September 2000   Volume 15, Number 3   ISBN 1-56053-327-7

OCCUPATIONAL MEDICINE: State of the Art Reviews is published quarterly by Hanley & Belfus, Inc., 210 South 13th Street, Philadelphia, Pennsylvania 19107. Periodical postage paid at Philadelphia, PA, and at additional mailing offices.

POSTMASTER: Send address changes to OCCUPATIONAL MEDICINE: State of the Art Reviews, Hanley & Belfus, Inc., 210 South 13th Street, Philadelphia, PA 19107.

The 2000 subscription price is $96.00 per year U.S., $106.00 outside U.S. (add $40.00 for air mail).

Occupational Medicine: State of the Art Reviews
Vol. 15, No. 3, July–September 2000

MULTIPLE CHEMICAL SENSITIVITY/IDIOPATHIC
ENVIRONMENTAL INTOLERANCE
Patricia J. Sparks, MD, Editor

CONTENTS

Idiopathic Environmental Intolerances: Overview **497**
Patricia J. Sparks

The editor discusses usage of the terms "idiopathic environmental intolerance," "multiple chemical sensitivity," and "environmental illness." Also addressed are prevalence, theories of etiology, evaluation and treatment, and social and political implications. **Occup Med 15:497–510, 2000**

Idiopathic Environmental Intolerance: Case Definition Issues. **511**
Richard Kreutzer

Case definitions of the same phenomenon may be different for different purposes. Case definitions usually become more specific over time as more information about the condition becomes available. Idiopathic environmental intolerance is one of many labels for a heterogeneous group of conditions in which subjects describe multiple symptoms that are attributed to exposure to extremely low doses of common chemicals. Dr. Kreutzer presents issues in case definition for clinical purposes and for population-based studies, and makes recommendations for the clinician and for the public health investigator. **Occup Med 15:511–517, 2000**

Behavioral Conditioning and Idiopathic Environmental Intolerance **519**
Nicholas D. Giardino and Paul M. Lehrer

Idiopathic environmental intolerance (IEI) is a poorly understood condition that may involve disturbances in immunologic, neurologic, endocrine, behavioral, emotional, and cognitive processes. This chapter reviews theories and evidence that behavioral conditioning processes, including pharmacologic sensitization, conditioned immunomodulation, and conditioned odor and taste aversions, may play a role in the development and maintenance of IEI. It also reviews the psychophysiologic concepts of individual response specificity and situational response stereotypy as potential explanations for the individual differences observed in specific responses to environmental stimuli in patients with IEI. Finally, the treatment implications of a conditioning account of IEI are discussed as part of a more comprehensive treatment approach that incorporates other behavioral and nonbehavioral strategies. **Occup Med 15:519–528, 2000**

**Idiopathic Environmental Intolerances: Results of
Challenge Studies.** **529**
Arthur Leznoff and Karen E. Binkley

It has been postulated that psychophysiologic mechanisms may account for symptom generation in IEI. In this review, the similarity of IEI and panic disorder symptoms are noted. The results of various challenge studies, both with known panicogenic substances and self-identified triggers, are examined. Available data are consistent with the premise that IEI symptoms have a psychophysiologic basis. **Occup Med 15:529–537, 2000**

Chemosensory Function and Response in Idiopathic Environmental Intolerance 539
Pamela Dalton and Thomas Hummel

This chapter reviews the current literature on the possible role of olfactory and trigeminal chemosensory function in idiopathic environmental intolerances (IEI). Two general points emerge from the review. First, studies of chemosensory function in IEI patients indicate that, despite their self-reported "heightened sensitivity" and enhanced responsivity to environmental odors, when compared to healthy controls they generally are found to be equally or even less sensitive to odors as measured by objective psychophysical and electrophysiological measures of olfactory function. These studies point towards alterations in the cognitive processing of olfactory information as the major characteristic of IEI. Second, studies of the role of sensitivity and bias in olfactory and trigeminal chemosensory functioning indicate that nonsensory factors (e.g., attention, bias, personality) can dramatically alter the self-reported impact of exposure to volatile chemicals. Together, these general points suggest a perspective on IEI that views many symptoms of the disorder to primarily reflect the influence of nonsensory, cognitive processes on responses to environmental odors. **Occup Med 15:539–556, 2000**

The Relationship of Mental Disorders and Idiopathic Environmental Intolerance 557
Donald W. Black

Idiopathic environmental intolerance (IEI) is an acquired condition with multiple symptoms associated with diverse environmental factors tolerated by most persons, not explained by known medical or psychiatric disorders. Data from clinical and epidemiologic samples show a robust association between IEI and lifetime psychiatric disorder, particularly mood, anxiety, somatoform, and personality disorders. IEI has *not* been associated with lifetime substance use disorders or psychotic disorders. The relationship of IEI and psychiatric disorder is important to acknowledge because it alerts clinicians to the fact that many persons diagnosed with IEI suffer treatable emotional illnesses, and because it suggests that some persons with mental illness are being misdiagnosed when their symptoms are misinterpreted as evidence of IEI. **Occup Med 15:557–570, 2000**

Sick Building Syndrome 571
Michael Hodgson

Dr. Hodgson summarizes what is known about human symptoms and discomfort in the built environment, and formulates several critical hypotheses that show striking parallels to the questions arising from discussions of the IEI/MCS syndrome. **Occup Med 15:571–585, 2000**

Chemical Sensitivity and Gulf War Veterans' Illnesses 587
Susan P. Proctor

Dr. Proctor summarizes the current research literature describing Gulf War (GW) veterans' health issues, particularly as they pertain to chemical sensitivity (CS) and multiple chemical sensitivity (MCS) syndrome. In several studies of GW veterans, using differing criteria and varying assessment measures for CS and MCS, the prevalence rates for CS are reported to be 36–86% in Department of Veterans' Affairs patient populations and 0.8–20% in general cohorts of GW veterans. The rates of MCS are 2–6%. Targeted research is needed to adequately evaluate GW veterans' health concerns and MCS. **Occup Med 15:587–599, 2000**

Diagnostic Evaluation and Treatment of the Patient Presenting with Idiopathic Environmental Intolerance **601**
Patricia J. Sparks

This chapter addresses the diagnostic evaluation and treatment of the patient presenting with idiopathic environmental intolerance (IEI). Clinicians with different views about the pathogenesis of IEI may agree on clinical management programs aimed at improved symptom control and functional ability. **Occup Med 15:601–609, 2000**

Functional Brain Imaging in the Assessment of Multiple Chemical Sensitivities **611**
Alan D. Waxman

The author provides a brief overview of single photon emission computed tomography in the assessment of multiple chemical sensitivities. **Occup Med 15:611–616, 2000**

Use of Neuropsychological Testing in Idiopathic Environmental Testing .. **617**
Karen I. Bolla

Individuals with idiopathic environmental intolerance (IEI) report fatigue, headaches, weakness, malaise, decreased attention/concentration, memory loss, disorientation, confusion, and psychological disturbances. These neurobehavioral symptoms may be a sign of possible alterations in the central nervous system (CNS). The evaluation of neurobehavioral functioning using standardized testing provides a surrogate measure of integrity of the CNS. However, the interpretation of neuropsychological test results must be made cautiously since this technique is extremely sensitive, but not specific. Abnormal test results could be due to a neurological disorder, a medical disorder, or a neuropsychiatric disorder. Therefore, when evaluating patients who present with symptoms of IEI, abnormal neurobehavioral results should not be attributed routinely to environmental chemical exposure until other causes are systematically ruled out. **Occup Med 15:617–625, 2000**

Psychological Treatment of Psychogenic Idiopathic Environmental Intolerance **627**
Herman Staudenmayer

This chapter focuses on the psychotherapy of individuals who suffer distress from functional somatic syndromes; specifically, idiopathic environmental intolerance (IEI). While patients believe environmental intolerances cause their distress, its origin is treated as psychological, mediated through psychophysiological systems and mechanisms associated with the stress response. Factors considered include stress and trauma premorbid to the alleged onset of IEI; somatization and its expression through affective, anxiety, and somatoform disorders; personality disorders and associated psychological defenses; motivation for the sick role; and iatrogenic suggestion and reinforcement of unsubstantiated toxicogenic theories and treatments. Psychotherapies include behavioral desensitization, cognitive-behavioral therapy, cognitive therapy, and psychotropic medications. The greatest challenge in treatment is to overcome the patient's disabling belief in a toxicogenic explanation for his or her symptoms. **Occup Med 15:627–646, 2000**

Immunologic Parameters of Multiple Chemical Sensitivity............. **647**
Clifford S. Mitchell, Albert Donnay, Donald R. Hoover, and
Joseph B. Margolick

Immunologic abnormalities have long been advanced as a potential mechanism for
multiple chemical sensitivity (MCS). An immunologic mechanism is supported in
part by the systemic nature of the symptoms reported, the complex interactions
known to exist between the immune system and other systems, and limited experimental evidence. However, there are both theoretical grounds for doubting an immunologic mechanism in MCS and methodological constraints in many of the
studies that have been conducted in humans. The authors discuss the structure and
function of the immune system as it potentially applies to MCS, the uses and limitations of immunologic testing, and the evidence for immunologic theories of
MCS. They describe recent work to validate some of the immunologic tests used in
MCS and consider opportunities for further research. **Occup Med 15:647–665,
2000**

Index **667**

CONTRIBUTORS

Karen E. Binkley, MD, FRCPC
Assistant Professor, Division of Clinical Immunology, Department of Medicine, University of Toronto, Toronto, Ontario, Canada

Donald W. Black, MD
Psychiatry Research, University of Iowa College of Medicine, Iowa City, Iowa

Karen I. Bolla, PhD
Associate Professor, Department of Neurology, Division of Occupational Medicine, Johns Hopkins Medical Institutions, Baltimore, Maryland

Pamela Dalton, PhD
Monell Chemical Senses Center, Philadelphia, Pennsylvania

Albert Donnay, MHS
President, MCS Referral & Resources, Baltimore, Maryland

Nicholas D. Giardino, MS
Graduate Student (PhD Candidate), Department of Psychology, Rutgers–The State University of New Jersey, Piscataway, New Jersey

Michael Hodgson, MD, MPH
National Institute of Occupational Safety and Health, Washington DC

Donald R. Hoover, PhD
Associate Professor, Department of Statistics, Rutgers–The State University of New Jersey, Piscataway, New Jersey

Thomas Hummel, MD
Department of Otorhinolaryngology, University of Dresden, Dresden, Germany

Richard A. Kreutzer, MD
Chief, Environmental Health Investigations Branch, California Department of Health Services, Oakland, California

Paul M. Lehrer, PhD
Professor, Department of Psychiatry, University of Medicine and Dentistry–Robert Wood Johnson Medical School, Piscataway, New Jersey

Arthur Leznoff, MD, FRCP(C)
Associate Professor, Department of Medicine, University of Toronto, Toronto, Ontario, Canada

Joseph B. Margolick, MD, PhD
Professor, Departments of Molecular Microbiology and Immunology, Environmental Health, and Epidemiology, Johns Hopkins University School of Hygiene and Public Health, Baltimore, Maryland

Clifford S. Mitchell, MD, MPH
Assistant Professor, Department of Environmental Health Sciences, Division of Occupational and Environmental Health, Johns Hopkins University School of Hygiene and Public Health, Baltimore, Maryland

Susan P. Proctor, DSc
Research Associate Professor, Department of Environmental Health, Boston University School of Public Health, and Department of Neurology, Boston University School of Medicine; Assistant Director, Boston Environmental Hazards Center, VA Boston Healthcare System; Research Associate, Women's Health Sciences Division, National Center for Post-Traumatic Stress Disorder, VA Boston Healthcare System, Boston, Massachusetts

Patricia J. Sparks, MD, MPH
Private Consultant, Occupational and Environmental Medicine, Mercer Island, Washington

Herman Staudenmayer, PhD
Behavioral Medicine and Biofeedback Clinic of Denver, Denver, Colorado

Alan D. Waxman, MD
Department of Imaging and Nuclear Medicine, Cedars-Sinai Medical Center, Los Angeles, California

PREFACE

The purpose of this book is to present recent research data and practical clinical information regarding idiopathic environmental intolerance (also known as multiple chemical sensitivity) and related issues such as Gulf War syndrome and sick building syndrome. The chapters were selected to reflect the most robust research data pertaining to the major theories regarding etiology, evaluation, and treatment of these syndromes.

Patricia J. Sparks, MD
EDITOR

PUBLISHED ISSUES
(available from the publisher)

January 1991   **Prevention of Pulmonary Disease in the Workplace**
Philip Harber and John R. Balmes, Editors

April 1991   **The Biotechnology Industry**
Alan M. Ducatman and Daniel F. Liberman, Editors

July 1991   **Health Hazards of Farming**
D. H. Cordes and Dorothy Foster Rea, Editors

October 1991   **The Nuclear Energy Industry**   Gregg S. Wilkinson, Editor

January 1992   **Back School Programs**   Lynne A. White, Editor

April 1992   **Occupational Lung Disease**
William S. Beckett and Rebecca Bascom, Editors

July 1992   **Unusual Occupational Diseases**
Dennis J. Shusterman and Paul D. Blanc, Editors

October 1992   **Ergonomics**   J. Steven Moore and Arun Garg, Editors

January 1993   **The Mining Industry**   Daniel E. Banks, Editor

April 1993   **Spirometry**   Ellen A. Eisen, Editor

July 1993   **De Novo Toxicants**   Dennis J. Shusterman and Jack E. Peterson, Editors

October 1993   **Women Workers**   Dana M. Headapohl, Editor

January 1994   **Occupational Skin Disease**   James R. Nethercott, Editor

April 1994   **Safety and Health Training**   Michael J. Colligan, Editor

July 1994   **Reproductive Hazards**
Ellen B. Gold, B. L. Lasley, and Marc B. Schenker, Editors

October 1994   **Tuberculosis in the Workplace**   Steven Markowitz, Editor

January 1995   **Effects of the Indoor Environment on Health**
James M. Seltzer, Editor

April 1995   **Construction Safety and Health**
Knut Ringen, Laura Welch, James L. Weeks, Jane L. Seegal,
and Anders Englund, Editors

July 1995   **Occupational Hearing Loss**
Thais C. Morata and Derek E. Dunn, Editors

October 1995   **Firefighters' Safety and Health**
Peter Orris, Richard M. Duffy, and James Melius, Editors

January 1996   **Law and the Workplace**
Jack W. Snyder and Julia E. Klees, Editors

April 1996   **Violence in the Workplace**   Robert Harrison, Editor

July 1996   **Occupational Epidemiology**   Ki Moon Bang, Editor

October 1996   **Psychosocial and Corporate Issues in Occupational Dysfunction**
Ibrahim Farid and Carroll Brodsky, Editors

January 1997   **The Pharmaceutical Industry**   Gregg M. Stave and Ron Joines, Editors

April 1997   **Human Health Effects of Pesticides**   Matthew C. Keifer, Editor

July 1997   **Diagnostic Testing**   Michael H. LeWitt, Editor

October 1997   **The Health Care Worker**
Melissa A. McDiarmid and Ellen Kessler, Editors

2000 ISSUES

The Workplace and Cardiovascular Disease
Edited by Peter Schnall, MD, MPH
and Dean Baker, MD, MPH
University of California, Irvine, California;
Paul Landsbergis, PhD, EdD, MPH
Cornell University, New York, New York;
Karen Belkić, MD, PhD
University of Southern California
Los Angeles, California

Occupational Asthma
Edited by Daniel E. Banks, MD
and Mei-Lin Wang, MD
West Virginia University
Morgantown, West Virginia

Multiple Chemical Sensitivity/ Idiopathic Environmental Intolerance
Edited by Patricia J. Sparks, MD, MPH
Private Consultant
Occupational and Environmental
    Medicine
Mercer Island, Washington

Risk and Disability Evaluation in the Workplace
Edited by David C. Randolph, MD, MPH
Occupational Medicine Physician
    and Consultant
Private Practice
Cincinnatti, Ohio

1999 ISSUES

Office Ergonomics
Edited by Martin Cherniack, MD, MPH
University of Connecticut
Farmington, Connecticut

Animal Handlers
Edited by Ricky L. Langley, MD, MPH
North Carolina Department of Health
    and Human Services
Raleigh, North Carolina

Special Populations
Edited by Howard Frumkin, MD
Emory University, Atlanta, Georgia
and Glenn Pransky, MD, MOccH
University of Massachusetts
Worcester, Massachusetts

Health Issues in the Plastics and Rubber Industries
Edited by Richard Lewis, MD, MPH
University of Louisville,
Louisville, Kentucky

1998 ISSUES

Low Back Pain
Edited by Gerard A. Malanga, MD
University of Medicine and Dentistry
    of New Jersey
Newark, New Jersey

Workers' Compensation
Edited by T. L. Guidotti, MD, MPH
University of Alberta
Edmonton, Alberta, Canada
and John W. F. Cowell, MD, Msc
Workers' Compensation Board of Alberta
Edmonton, Alberta, Canada

Hand and Upper Extremity Injuries
Edited by Morton L. Kasdan, MD
University of Louisville
Louisville, Kentucky
and V. Jane Derebery, MD
Concentra Medical Center
Austin Texas

Managed Care
Edited by Jeffrey S. Harris, MD, MPH, MBA
J. Harris Associates, Inc.
Mill Valley, California

Ordering Information:
Subscriptions for full year and single issues are available from the publishers—
Hanley & Belfus, Inc., 210 South 13th Street, Philadelphia, PA 19107
Telephone (215) 546-7293; (800) 962-1892. Fax (215) 790-9330. Website www.hanleyandbelfus.com

PATRICIA J. SPARKS, M.D., M.P.H.

IDIOPATHIC ENVIRONMENTAL INTOLERANCES: OVERVIEW

From Private Practice
Occupational and Environmental
   Medicine and Clinical Toxicology
Mercer Island, Washington

Reprint requests to:
Patricia J. Sparks, M.D., M.P.H.
7683 SE 27th Street
Mercer Island, WA 98040

Idiopathic environmental illness (IEI) is defined as an acquired disorder with multiple recurrent symptoms, associated with diverse environmental factors tolerated by the majority of people, and not explained by any known medical or psychiatric disorder.[38]

The name IEI supplants, and is more inclusive than, other terms such as multiple chemical sensitivity (MCS) syndrome and environmental illness (EI). The term IEI also attempts to address other of the numerous, ever-shifting labels assigned to patients reporting symptoms they attribute to environmental exposure according to the most recent hypothesis regarding etiology.

A select panel convened by the World Health Organization[38] concluded that the MCS and EI labels should be replaced for several reasons: (1) Use of the word "sensitivity" in a diagnostic label can be construed as connoting an allergic or other idiosyncratic pathophysiologic cause of these phenomena, and there is no scientific foundation for such causative explanations. (2) Environmental intolerances other than chemicals have been described (for example, electromagnetic fields). (3) The relationship between symptoms and putative exposures is unproven. (4) Neither MCS nor EI can be recognized as a clinically defined disease with generally accepted underlying pathophysiologic mechanisms or validated criteria for diagnosis.

The use of the term IEI in this volume is meant to encompass those syndromes previously labeled as MCS or EI, as well as similar aspects of other phenomena included in such labels as "sick building syndrome" and "Gulf War syndrome."

IEI must be distinguished from objectively defined illness and injury diagnoses, such as allergic rhinitis/sinusitis or asthma. In these conditions, objective findings are present during active disease, and the causal relationship of those findings to environmental exposure is more readily established. In clinical practice, however, there may be overlap between acute and chronic occupational or environmental illnesses such as asthma, associated with objective signs of disease, and IEI.

There have been attempts to define IEI for clinical and research purposes. In this volume, Kreutzer notes that case definitions for IEI may be used for different purposes, including clinical diagnosis and population-based studies and investigation. Differing case definitions used in most studies hamper estimations of prevalence and comparisons across studies. Nevertheless, even in the absence of a case definition, population studies still can be performed, and form the basis for further clinical research.

This volume represents a compilation of recent research data pertaining to the etiology, evaluation, and treatment of IEI. It is not a comprehensive review, but rather focus was given to human research elucidating potential causal mechanisms and contributing to clinical management of these patients. The reader is referred to comprehensive reviews for a more complete discussion of etiologic theories.[63,64,35]

Other chapters here discuss sick building syndrome and Gulf War syndrome as each pertain to IEI. It is noted that these two phenomena are not the same as IEI, but there are overlapping features. Also, a high percentage of patients labeled with other subjectively defined syndromes, such as fibromyalgia and chronic fatigue syndrome, report symptoms consistent with IEI.[15]

PREVALENCE

It is difficult to assess the prevalence of a condition with a variable, subjectively defined case definition without validated objective findings. Although definitive population-based studies have not been published, the estimated prevalence of IEI is 0.2–4% of the general population in the United States.[15] Women represent 70–80% of the affected population. No published population prevalence estimates are available for the United Kingdom or other European populations, or for developing countries.[35]

A survey of the self-reported prevalence of allergy and chemical sensitivity in a rural population in eastern North Carolina found that chemical sensitivity was reported by 33% of individuals, with 18.3% reporting symptoms from chemical sensitivity at least once or more each week; 3.9% of the population reported symptoms almost daily.[49] There is a report of varying severity of self-reported chemical odor intolerance in 15–30% of college student and active, retired, elderly populations.[12,13]

A telephone survey performed by the California Department of Health$_1$ found that 6.3% of those surveyed had been given a diagnosis of EI or MCS, and 15.9% considered themselves allergic or unusually sensitive to everyday chemicals such as household cleaners, paints, perfumes, and soaps. About 3% considered themselves restricted in activities of daily living because of their sensitivities.

Many IEI patients (about 40%) report the onset of symptoms as being gradual, with no specific exposure or event recalled. Across various studies the most prevalent symptoms have involved the central nervous system, respiratory system, and gastrointestinal tract—although symptoms in all organ systems have been reported, and there is no consistent pattern of symptoms that distinguishes patients with IEI from those labeled with other diagnoses manifested primarily by subjective symptoms.

Almost any environmental exposure has been described to precipitate symptoms. No single chemical exposure or psychosocial situation appears to have been more prevalent than any other in association with the onset of IEI.[31]

THEORIES OF ETIOLOGY OF IEI

A broad spectrum of individuals may be diagnosed with IEI. As most physicians only see a few of these patients who are quite heterogeneous, caution is recommended in generalizing experience with one patient to others with this diagnosis; the condition may not represent a single clinical entity.

There are four major views about the etiology of this syndrome, although more than one of these proposed mechanisms are likely to be operating in different patients, and there is some overlap among the views of pathogenesis. One view is that IEI is a primarily physical or toxicological reaction to multiple environmental chemical exposures. A second view is that IEI symptoms may be precipitated by low-level environmental exposures, but the underlying increased sensitivity is due primarily to psychophysiologic factors or stress, such that IEI is primarily a behavioral phenomenon. A third view is that IEI is a misdiagnosis, and chemical exposure is not the cause of the symptoms. In this case, the symptoms may be due to misdiagnosed physical or psychological illness. The fourth view is that IEI is simply a culturally acquired belief system instilled by certain practitioners, the media, or others in society; IEI is therefore the manifestation of culturally shaped illness behavior. These theories are discussed in more detail elsewhere.[63,34,35] This chapter focuses on theories of etiology for which the data is the most robust in humans.

Physical/Toxicological Mechanisms

Assuming that symptoms in IEI may be caused by environmental exposure (predominately to synthetic chemicals), proposed causal mechanisms include immunologic injury, nonspecific neurogenic inflammation of the respiratory tract, and neurotoxicity.

IMMUNOLOGIC THEORIES

The concept of "allergy" has been invoked as a rationale for why IEI patients experience symptoms on exposure to various chemical substances at doses far lower than those associated with objective manifestations of toxicity in most similarly exposed individuals. The immunologic theory has received much attention in the past based on case reports,[22,68,44,70] and research has accumulated more recently in well-designed controlled studies.

Simon[59] performed a controlled and blinded study of IEI clinic patients and controls selected from a musculoskeletal clinic population. There were no significant differences between cases and controls in the prevalence of "positive" anti-tissue, autoimmune antibodies or anti-chemical antibodies; the average number of T-cell lymphocyte subsets (including TA1 cells); or the generation of interleukin-1 by in vitro cultured monocytes. Immunologic assays generally have shown poor reproducibility during submission of duplicate samples to a commercial laboratory. Methodological problems were suggested when, on a limited number of split samples, the reliability of the laboratory was little better than chance.

Margolik[45] studied both cellular and humoral immune parameters in MCS in two phases. The first phase was designed to establish a mechanism for obtaining reliable immunologic measurements on people with MCS and control populations. The second phase was a rigorous, detailed comparison of whether any of the tests selected distinguished between people with MCS and people with other chronic illnesses or no illness. Margolik found that the tests performed by the participating laboratories were sufficiently reliable to find substantial differences between MCS patients and other groups if such differences existed. The second phase emphasized comparisons between the group with MCS and the healthy control group. Although subtle differences in T cell subsets between the two groups were found, these differences were not thought to be of clinical or diagnostic significance. The autoantibodies studied showed little difference between the two groups. The authors concluded that, taken as a whole, the data do not support the use of any of the immunological tests as a diagnostic tool for MCS.

The proper interpretation of any laboratory test must rely on how well the test discriminates between patients with and without the disease, and what impact the test result has on clinical decision-making.[69] No controlled and blinded challenge studies have been published demonstrating a consistent pattern of alteration in immune parameters in IEI patients following chemical exposure, even with the patient serving as his or her own control. Even if immunologic changes were to be subsequently confirmed, their role with regard to IEI is not clear. There has been no attempt to relate a particular set of symptoms and/or exposures to any specific alteration in function. The lack of consistency in response patterns both between and within individual patients with IEI argues against this theory.[35]

THEORIES OF NONSPECIFIC INFLAMMATION

Other investigators have postulated that IEI is related, at least in part, to altered function of the respiratory mucosa through amplification of the nonspecific immune response to low-level irritants.[8,9,51] It has been postulated that symptoms might be mediated through c-fiber neurons and the release by the airway epithelium of cytokines, producing an acute local inflammatory response or altered neuroepithelial interaction. Sensory c-fibers may serve as both afferent and efferent nerves for neurogenic inflammation triggered by environmental irritants and may release various mediators, such as substance P, capable of producing vasodialation, edema, and other manifestations of inflammation. Substance P is degraded by neutral endopeptidase (NEP) whose action is inhibited by environmental irritants such as cigarette smoke. It is postulated that depletion of NEP or other enzymes by irritant exposure might amplify the response to exposure to other irritants.

One study[48] described findings of edema, excessive mucus, a cobblestone appearance of the posterior pharynx and base of the tongue, focal areas of blanched mucosa, and mucosal injection in 10 IEI patients who underwent rhinolaryngoscopy. In a preliminary study of a small number patients who developed IEI in temporal association with an irritant exposure, upper airway biopsies revealed defects in tight junctions, mucosal desquamation, glandular hyperplasia, lymphocytic infiltrates, and peripheral nerve fiber proliferation.[49] A model is proposed in which a positive feedback loop is set up between the inflammatory response to low-level irritants and the epithelial changes produced by the inflammation.[51]

Studies of exposure to the organic vapor phase of environmental tobacco smoke (ETS) in rats have demonstrated vascular extravasation of inflammatory mediators thought to occur from irritant stimulation of the c-fiber neurons.[43] Bascom has shown that this response does not appear to occur in humans. However, vascular congestion due to vasodialation appears to be the mechanism of increased nasal resistance observed in human subjects with self-reported sensitivity to ETS when challenged with brief high levels of tobacco smoke.[7,10] An increase in baseline nasal resistance in response to odors also has been observed in patients with IEI when compared to controls.[10,30]

Some of the findings, presented by Bascomb at a recent meeting, have not yet been published or replicated, but do suggest that the upper respiratory tract may well play a major role in mediating at least some of the common airway symptoms in patients with IEI.[10] Bascomb challenged subjects complaining of ETS sensitivity with ETS and noted an acute increase in nasal resistance compared to normal controls (but no delayed response as is seen in the lower respiratory tract). Those showing an increase in nasal resistance also were more sensitive to substance P (produced by c-fibers). To test whether a deficit of airway surface fluid might be playing a role in ETS sensitivity, Bascomb has been able to demonstrate a more blunted mucocilliary clearance response to ETS in sensitive subjects compared to normal controls. In animals, mucociliary clearance is increased at low doses and is blunted at higher doses of exposure to irritants. This led to the hypothesis that sensitive subjects may have an altered dose-response curve. Bascom also noted that airway surface fluid may be altered by the presentation of antigen in allergic subjects prior to exposure to ETS.

Neurogenic inflammation of the upper respiratory tract does not appear to account for all the multiorgan system complaints in IEI patients, but might help explain some of them, in some patients.

NEUROTOXIC THEORIES

One theory of causation of IEI proposes a biologic mechanism, with much overlap with the behavior conditioning model and the primary psychiatric illness models described below. It has been proposed that chemical sensitivity may be a neural sensitization phenomenon: exposure to odors and respiratory irritants may precipitate physiologic and psychological symptoms, due to interactions between the nervous (limbic) and endocrine systems.[16,61] A recent review from the United Kingdom cited this theory as one of the most plausible explanations for IEI that requires further investigation.[35]

There are direct anatomic links between the olfactory nerve, the limbic system (including portions of the hippocampus, amygdala, cingulate, and subcallosal gyri), and the hypothalamus, which govern the parasympathetic and sympathetic nervous systems. Bell postulates that these rich neural interconnections may explain how odor or irritation of the respiratory tract indirectly produces symptoms referable to multiple organ systems.[16]

Most of the data cited to support this theory are indirect in humans or from animal studies. Rodent studies[32] show that single, high-level or intermittently repeated, low-level environmental chemical exposures cause **limbic kindling**. Kindling is defined as the ability of a repeated, intermittent electrical or chemical stimulus that is initially incapable of producing a response to eventually induce seizure activity in later applications. Animal studies also demonstrate **time-dependent sensitization**, which is the amplification of subsequent responses to a chemical or novel and threatening psychological stimulus by the passage of time between stimuli.[6]

It has been suggested[11,14,16,61] that subconvulsive chemical kindling of the olfactory bulb, amygdala, piriform cortex, and hippocampus, as well as time-dependent sensitization (TDS), are central nervous system mechanisms that could amplify reactivity and lower the threshold of response to low levels of inhaled chemicals. Low-level inhaled chemicals could initiate persistent affective, cognitive, and somatic symptomatology in some vulnerable individuals who may be genetically predisposed to affective spectrum disorders (such as panic disorder and depression). This neurologic sensitization might occur either with a single, high-dose exposure to a chemical substance, followed by much smaller subtoxic levels of exposure to the same chemical, or with repeated, lower-dose exposures, as has been demonstrated in animals.[15]

Kindling and time-dependent sensitization may explain the initiation in some individuals of psychiatric disorders such as depression[54] and post-traumatic stress disorder[52] independently of the IEI phenomenon. Further, they suggest some commonality in the causal mechanisms for these psychiatric disorders and IEI in some patients. Bell emphasizes that sensitization is distinct, although interactive with other psychological mechanisms (e.g., behavioral conditioning) which may occur simultaneously.[16]

There are, however, no experimental data in humans to support or refute the role of chemically induced kindling or TDS in producing IEI, or to determine whether the proposed mechanisms, if verified experimentally, would be specific to IEI patients. In addition, kindling occurs in animals in response to pharmacologically effective doses of drugs or other chemical substances rather than trace exposures. Finally, the proposed effects of TDS in humans may be indistinguishable from those that are behaviorally or cognitively mediated. At present this theory has not been experimentally or epidemiologically separated from the theories of primary psychological origin of illness in IEI (see chapters here by Giardino and Lehrer, Black, and Staudenmayer).

There is limited peer-reviewed literature with regard to neurotoxicity and abnormalities on functional brain imaging. The studies that have been published have had poor study design with lack of appropriate controls or validation of findings.[60]

Brain imaging technology, including SPECT, has been applied to IEI patients and patients with chronic fatigue syndrome[36] (see chapter here by Waxman). This study used both computerized quantitative methods and qualitative visual methods on all study participants. It demonstrated nonspecific differences in global perfusion and in the ventricular and anterior cingulate regions of the brain in IEI patients compared to normal and CFS patients using the quantitative technique. The findings could not conclusively distinguish the SPECT findings of IEI cases from patients with anxiety, depression, or obsessive-compulsive disorders. Unfortunately, there is no diagnostic gold-standard or tissue pathology to validate findings in IEI patients. The study used a computerized quantitative method to develop a discriminant function for distinguishing IEI cases from controls. Few differences could be distinguished by the visual methods of analysis used in most laboratories.

At this time, no controlled and blinded studies have demonstrated any patterns of abnormalities on brain imaging studies (such as SPECT or PET scans) that would clearly distinguish IEI patients from normals or individuals with primary psychiatric disorders.

Tests of **neuropsychological function** in IEI[31,59] found that IEI patients differed little from controls on selected measures, despite the high prevalence of complaints of cognitive dysfunction (see Bolla's chapter here). There are no data that IEI patients demonstrate a consistent or specific pattern of neurocognitive deficits, at least in cross-sectional studies, and disturbances of memory and attention observed in some IEI patients may be a result of depression and/or anxiety. The interpretation of neuropsychological test results must be made cautiously, as the technique is very sensitive, but not very specific. Abnormal test results could be due to a neurologic disorder, medical disorder, or a neuropsychiatric disorder. Abnormal neurobehavioral results should not be attributed routinely to environmental chemical exposure until other causes are systematically ruled out.

The relationship of IEI symptoms to environmental chemical exposures does not appear to fit established principles of toxicology. The intensity of exposure to various chemical exposures does not correlate with the prevalence of IEI symptoms, violating a basic tenet of toxicology: "The dose makes the poison." There is agreement among occupational health professionals that any natural or synthetic chemical exposure in sufficient doses may be harmful to specific organs of the body and can produce objectively measurable toxic effects. Causal relationships between toxic exposures and human disease generally are established by determining the strength of the association between exposure and the development of disease using epidemiological methods and toxicologic animal models, dose-response relationships, and the consistency and predictability of the clinical responses to specific chemical exposures in affected human subjects.[66] In IEI, all of these criteria are lacking. Still, one must keep an open mind to the possibility that a different paradigm exists to explain the phenomenon of IEI.

IEI As a Behavioral Phenomenon

BEHAVIORAL CONDITIONING AND STRESS

Some investigators have proposed a behavioral conditioned response to odor,[20] in which a strong-smelling, chemical irritant causes a direct and unconditioned physical or psychophysiologic response. Later, the same odor or irritant at a much lower concentration causes a conditioned response of the same symptoms. Through stimulus generalization, different odors or irritants become the precipitant for similar symptoms.

Several conditioning-related phenomena, including pharmacological sensitization, conditioned immunomodulation, and odor and taste aversion, are examples of processes that may share some common features with IEI (see chapter here by Giardino and Lehrer). Individual response specificity and situational response specificity might explain individual differences in specific responses to environmental chemical exposures. Pavlovian conditioning does not entirely explain the wide array of symptoms presented by IEI patients. Also, in many cases of IEI there is no substantiated initial exposure event that would constitute the unconditioned stimulus. Nevertheless, human data on mechanisms of behavioral condition probably have relevance to some patients presenting with IEI.

There is research to support the hypothesis that the perceived risk of harm associated with an odor has a great deal to do with one's psychophysiologic reaction to the odor (see chapter here by Dalton and Hummel). Survey data has indicated that perceived risk from exposure was the most significant correlate of odor annoyance from factories with occasional emissions.[46] Dalton confirmed experimentally that there was a direct relationship between perceived risk and odor intensity.[27] Variation in perception and intensity of odors can result from the explicit characterization given to the odor, which gives support to the position that odor perception is both a sensory and cognitive function. Other studies have shown inhibition of olfactory adaptation and elevated olfactory sensitivity (hyperosmia) among individuals reporting high levels of anxiety or stress.[55,56]

The research of Dalton and Hummel suggests that while environmental factors may contribute to symptoms, cognitive, nonsensory factors play a major role in both the initiation and maintenance of IEI. Negative information about the consequences of exposure can elevate symptom reporting. The perception of health risk from short- or long-term exposure to volatile chemicals frequently is mediated by aware-ness of odors and/or irritation, and such concerns are likely to amplify the vigilance and attention paid to even low-level neutral or background odors.

There are small case series reports in which organic solvents[20,26,57] or cocaine[53] have precipitated panic attacks. Though there are limited data to support this con-tention, low-level exposure to irritants or odors may produce psychophysiologic symptoms which, in some vulnerable individuals, may evolve into IEI.

An exploration of the relationship between IEI and symptoms of anxiety has proved enlightening (see chapter by Leznoff and Binkley). Leznoff[41,42] challenged 15 IEI patients with trigger substances. The symptoms and signs were consistent with an anxiety reaction plus hyperventilation, and he proposes that IEI is a manifes-tation of an anxiety syndrome triggered by the perception of an environmental insult, with at least some symptoms induced by hyperventilation. Leznoff notes that one of the most common symptoms of IEI-impaired mentation often is described as "brain fog," which also is characteristic of acute hypocarbia caused by restriction of cerebral flow and decreased brain perfusion.

Binkley[17] reported on a study of patients referred to an allergy and clinical im-munology service for evaluation of "chemical sensitivity." After a standardized psy-chiatric assessment was performed, patients underwent single-blind intravenous infusion of a normal saline solution (placebo) and sodium lactate (which reproduces symptoms in individuals with underlying panic disorder). Four of the five patients met DSM-III-R diagnostic criteria for panic disorder, along with other depressive and/or anxiety related disorders. All five patients with self-identified chemical sensi-tivity exhibited a positive symptomatic response to sodium lactate compared with placebo infusion. The results suggest that IEI may have a neurobiologic basis simi-lar, if not identical, to that of panic disorder.

The concept of IEI as a type of phobic disturbance is compatible with a panic disorder hypothesis. Underlying panic disorder with conditioned phobic responses to "chemical" triggers could account for the full clinical picture in at least a subset of patients with IEI. Through the mechanism of conditioned response, environmen-tal "toxins" could become psychologically linked with panic symptoms. This link, reinforced by caregivers, could result in increased anticipatory anxiety, with produc-tion and maintenance of panic attacks and phobic avoidance—including reluctance to seek potentially helpful psychiatric treatments.[17]

IEI As Misdiagnosed Psychiatric Illness

It has been suggested that IEI is a misdiagnosis and chemical exposure is not the cause of the symptoms. In contrast, the patient's complaints may be due to a mis-diagnosed psychological illness. The likelihood of misdiagnosis may be fostered by conscious or subconscious attempts by the patient or physician to avoid a psychiatric diagnosis.[21,65,67,18] Research evidence in humans to support this theory is the most robust of all the theories we have discussed, with several caveats.

Published case series (with varying case definitions) have reported an increased frequency of symptoms categorized as depression, anxiety disorders, somatization, obsessive-compulsive disorder, and other personality disorders in persons diagnosed with IEI, as well as greater frequency of abnormal elevations on various psychologic symptom scales (see chapter here by Black).

In 1990, Black[18] compared 26 subjects recruited from a community and clinic population with IEI with 46 age- and sex-matched general population controls. Twenty-three were given standardized psychiatric assessments, including the

Diagnostic Interview Schedule (DIS) and the Structured Interview for DSM-III-R Personality Disorders. Several self-report instruments were used to assess somatic concerns, hypochondriacal behavior, and past and current major depression. Only three of the 23 subjects assessed were free of a major mental or personality disorder, a higher prevalence than community controls. The authors concluded that most patients diagnosed with environmental illness have unrecognized emotional problems that are not being appropriately diagnosed and treated. In this volume, Black presents follow-up data 9 years later on this same group of individuals, showing persistence of similar psychopathology.

Because of the possibility that IEI itself might produce psychiatric symptoms, some investigators have tried to evaluate the presence of preexisting symptoms of psychiatric illness in patients diagnosed with IEI.[58,59] Among the group of aerospace plastics workers evaluated by Sparks,[62] there was a subgroup of 13 who fit a case definition of IEI and who also had a history of decreased functional status due to their symptoms. A history of somatization and psychiatric morbidity predating workplace exposure to chemicals was the strongest predictor of IEI.[58]

Terr[67] found that the prior medical records of 90 patients diagnosed as having work-related IEI, and engaged in workers' compensation litigation, contained documented evidence of the same multiple symptoms for many years prior to the employment of concern in 56 (62%) of the cases.

Simon[59] evaluated psychological and other parameters in IEI, and included case and control groups from two defined clinic populations. The prevalence of a somatization symptom pattern among IEI patients prior to onset of IEI was significantly greater than in matched controls. While acknowledging that retrospective assessment has limited ability to discern temporal patterns of disease, the authors postulated that, among a substantial proportion of individuals who develop IEI, preexisting psychological vulnerability plays a significant role in the development of the syndrome.

The literature with regard to family history of individuals with IEI demonstrates significantly increased prevalence of mental illness (see Black's chapter). Moreover, individuals deployed during the Gulf War who exhibit symptoms of IEI have significantly increased prevalence of psychopathology prior to their being deployed or labeled with a diagnosis of IEI, MCS, or Gulf War syndrome. The overlap of these syndromes is discussed in Proctor's chapter in this volume.

Bell[16] and others have argued that one cannot exclude a common mechanism for the development of psychiatric illness and IEI. However, there is currently no data in humans that would establish the existence of a separate etiologic entity for IEI.

IEI As an Illness Belief System

In many ways, IEI is a belief system. Promoted by clinical ecologists and those sympathetic to their views, and followed by medically naive lay persons, the belief is reinforced by referring patients to a network of similarly minded clinicians, and establishing support groups, hotlines, journals, and clinics to support and reinforce these beliefs. Some have called this phenomenon a **medical subculture**. According to this model, the group psychosocial dynamic among patients diagnosed with IEI facilitates and perpetuates rationalizations regarding the role of external and uncontrollable factors in their illness. The model rejects the concept that symptoms are not indicative of severe disease or may have psychological components that can be helped by behavioral or pharmacological treatments. It promotes the assumption of the patient as a victim, associated with adversarial interactions with conventional healthcare and disability systems.[21]

IEI shares many features with other conditions, such as chronic fatigue syndrome, fibromyalgia, neurasthenia, sick building syndrome, and Gulf War syndrome, that encompass individuals with distress and functional disability characterized by few or no objective findings. It has been speculated that IEI is simply the most contemporary cultural expression of psychosomatic illness.[21] In at least some patients, IEI may result from iatrogenic (physician-induced) hypochondriasis.[19]

Some specific symptoms of IEI may be triggered by suggestion. In 1896, McKenzie[47] noted that a patient who was allergic to roses displayed an asthma reaction when presented with an artificial rose. The visual features of the rose served as a conditioned stimulus for the allergic response. In the asthma literature, a number of studies have provided evidence that psychogenic asthma attacks can occur even when a person simply thinks that exposure to an asthma trigger has occurred.[40] A double-blind placebo-controlled study on intranasal chemoreception in patients with IEI, in which chemosensory event-related potentials were used an objective measure of outcome, demonstrated that 20% of subjects responded regardless of the type of challenge, suggesting that these individuals were susceptible to nonspecific experimental manipulation.[37] Thus, some IEI patients may respond on the basis of belief that they have been exposed to something capable of eliciting symptoms, rather than conditioning.

The majority of IEI patients do not simulate their symptoms, nor do symptoms in most IEI patients result only from suggestion or shaping on the part of the culture or their physicians. However, in some cases, the attribution of symptoms to environmental chemical exposure is likely due to these factors.

Summary of Theories of Pathogenesis

The available evidence shows that patients diagnosed with IEI are heterogeneous, and that more than one causal mechanism may be operative in different cases. It is possible that preexisting or concurrent psychiatric illness, particular health belief models, and psychological stress may produce a vulnerable group of individuals who then develop a sensitivity to odors or low-level chemical irritants that occurs as a result of one or more of the above proposed mechanisms. None of the above views of etiology of IEI is universally accepted on the basis of substantial scientific evidence, although the evidence for psychiatric/cognitive theories of etiology appear the most robust.

EVALUATION AND TREATMENT

The fact that there is no agreement on any one etiology for most patients with IEI does not prevent clinicians from helping affected patients with their symptoms. Central neurophysiologic alterations due to exogenous chemical exposures might represent toxic injury or a maladaptive, but reversible, central nervous system response pattern such as behavioral conditioning. The treatment and lifestyle implications of these alternative response patterns are contradictory, since chemically induced injury would probably preclude further exposure to the suspect chemicals and would justify some physicians' recommendations for chemical avoidance. However, the latter response pattern might be amenable to readaptation through behavioral, cognitive, environmental, or even pharmacological interventions, with the goal of progressive resumption of normal activity. In this volume, emphasis is placed on the latter assumption (see recommendations for medical management in chapters by Sparks and Staudenmayer).

SOCIAL AND POLITICAL IMPLICATIONS
OF THE IEI PHENOMENON

The administrative recognition of IEI as an occupational or environmental illness may interfere with the objective study of this phenomenon as a clinical condition.[25,33] Recognition of this syndrome as an illness with potential to cause permanent disability could necessitate changes in healthcare coverage and delivery, awarding of workers' compensation benefits, and the regulation of chemicals in the workplace and the environment. There also are social implications for the increasing human and economic cost of disability. Establishing whether IEI is due to a behavioral or psychological response to perceived chemical toxicity or to a toxic or pathophysiologic effect of low-level exposure on organ systems is critical to these issues.[34]

There is current pressure to answer several questions of social policy regarding IEI. The first issue is whether compensation should be awarded for a condition that relies entirely on a patient's report of subjective symptoms for diagnosis, without an objective basis for confirming the diagnosis, rating its severity, or even determining that it is due to environmental exposure.

Second, how might the expanded recognition of the phenomenon of IEI impact regulation and exposure control? Should employers attempt to reduce specific chemical exposures or to investigate organizational factors that may put an individual in a workplace at risk of expressing this type of illness? At this point, there is no evidence that controlling exposure to chemical substances far below levels associated with known toxic or irritant effects has any positive impact on symptom expression or the natural history of IEI.

Third, there is the perceived need to regulate and control nontraditional, unproven medical practices, such as those promoted by clinical ecologists and other "environmental physicians," to limit potentially dangerous or misleading practices and iatrogenic chronic disability.

IEI appeals to the widespread fear of man-made chemicals as well as the distrust that the public has of science, medicine, technology, and government.[34] Society has a justifiable concern about the role that chemical pollution has played in environmental deterioration over the past century and the long-term implications for humans and other animal species.

Some believe or fear that the current controversy surrounding IEI is similar to that which existed several decades ago regarding asbestos-related lung disease, and that medical science simply has not yet found a way to causally link environmental chemical exposure with the illness or to measure the impairment and disability of patients given an IEI diagnosis. Physicians who question or are agnostic about IEI's relationship to workplace or environmental exposure, and those who have performed research to test the hypotheses of environmental attribution advocates, have been targeted by hostile attack from IEI support groups and others with an economic stake in the outcome of the debate: in some cases, they have even been removed from government jobs for the expression of their views.[29]

Several medical societies and other organizations have issued position statements expressing concern about the IEI diagnoses, misuse of diagnostic procedures, use of inappropriate treatment modalities, and the lack of scientific support for the alleged toxic effects of environmental (chemical) exposure in patients labeled with various IEI diagnoses. These have included the American Academy of Allergy and Immunology,[2] the American College of Physicians,[4] the America College of Occupational and Environmental Medicine,[3] the Council of Scientific Affairs of the American Medical Association,[5] and the California Medical Association. The World

Health Organization[38] and the International Society of Regulatory Toxicology and Pharmacology[38] have held symposia on the subject. The American Council on Science and Health[24] and the General Medical Council of Great Britain have published reports indicating the lack of scientific basis for the attribution of the IEI illness to environmental exposures.

These efforts have angered many IEI patients who view them as an attempt by mainstream medicine to negate the existence of IEI as an illness. Yet the controversy is not about whether IEI patients have "real" vs. simulated illness, but rather about whether the illness (which is accepted as present) is explained by toxicologic vs. behavioral effects of chemical exposure, or culturally shaped fear of environmental chemical exposure.

Despite the controversy and lack of general medical acceptance of this diagnosis, IEI may increasingly impact the total burden of chronic disability, much as low back pain and cumulative trauma disorders of the upper extremities do now. IEI patients make an average of 23 healthcare visits per year.[14] It would thus be appropriate to allocate research funds to obtain the data necessary to further medically define this condition and its relationship to environmental exposure, as well as its appropriate diagnostic evaluation and treatment, and to educate the public to assure that medical science plays a major role in the social policy decisions relating to IEI.

REFERENCES

1. Agency for Toxic Substances and Disease Registry: Evaluating individuals reporting sensitivities to multiple chemicals: Final report. Washington DC, U.S Department of Heatlh and Human Services, 1996.
2. American Academy of Allergy, Asthma and Immunology: Position Statement: Idiopathic Environmental Intolerances. J Allergy Clin Immunol 103:36–40, 1999.
3. American College of Occupational and Environmental Medicine: ACOEM statement about distinctions among indoor air quality, MCS, and ETS [position statement]. ACOEM Report H5-H7. ACOEM, Arlington Heights, IL, 1993.
4. American College of Physicians: Position statement: Clinical ecology. Ann Intern Med 111:168–178, 1989.
5. American Medical Association, Council on Scientific Affairs: Clinical ecology: Council report. JAMA 268:3465–3470, 1992.
6. Antelman SM, Kocan D, Knopf S, et al: One brief exposure to a psychological stressor induces long-lasting, time-dependent sensitization of both the cataleptic and neurochemical responses to haloperidol. Life Sci 51:261–266, 1992.
7. Bascomb R, Kulle T, Kagey-Sobotka A, Proud D: Upper respiratory tract environmental tobacco smoke sensitivity. Am Rev Respir Dis 143:1304–1311, 1991.
8. Bascomb R: Multiple chemical sensitivity: A respiratory disorder? Toxicol Ind Health 8:221–228, 1992.
9. Bascomb R, Meggs W, Frampton M, et al: Neurogenic inflammation with additional discussion of central and perceptual integration in non-neurogenic inflammation. Environ Health Perspect 105(suppl 2):531–537, 1997.
10. Bascomb R: Differential responses to irritant exposure. Low-level environmental exposures: A state of the science update. Arlington, Virginia, Environmental Sensitivities Research Institute, 1999.
11. Bell IR, Miller CS, Schwartz GE: An olfactory-limbic model of multiple chemical sensitivity syndrome: Possible relationships to kindling and affective spectrum disorders. Biol Psychiatry 32:218–242, 1992.
12. Bell IR, Schwartz GE, Peterson JM, Amend D: Self-reported illness from chemical odors in young adults without clinical syndromes or occupational exposures. Arch Environ Health 48:6-13, 1993.
13. Bell IR, Schwartz GE, Peterson JM, et al: Possible time-dependent sensitization to xenobiotics: Self-reported illness from chemical odors, foods, and opiate drugs in an older adult population. Arch Environ Health 48(5):315–327, 1993.
14. Bell IR, Schwartz GE, Baldwin CM, et al: Individual differences in neural sensitization and the role of context in illness from low-level environmental chemical exposures. Environ Health Perspect 105(Suppl2),457–466, 1997.

15. Bell IR, Baldwin CM, Schwartz GE: Illness from low-level environmental chemicals: Relevance to chronic fatigue syndrome and fibromyalgia. Am J Med 105(3A):74S–82S, 1998.
16. Bell IR, Baldwin CM, Fernandez M, Schwartz GER: Neural sensitization model for multiple chemical sensitivity: Overview of theory and empirical evidence. Tox Ind Health 15(3-4):294–304, 1999.
17. Binkley KE, Krutcher S: Panic response to sodium lactate infusion in patients with multiple chemical sensitivity syndrome. J Allergy Clin Immunol 99(4):570–574, 1997.
18. Black DW, Rathe A, Goldstein RB: Environmental illness: A controlled study of 26 subjects with 20th century disease. JAMA 264:3166–3170, 1990.
19. Black DW: Iatrogenic (physician-induced) hypochondriasis: Four patient examples of "chemical sensitivity." Psychosomatics 37:390–393, 1996.
20. Bolla-Wilson K, Wilson RJ, Bleecker ML: Conditioning of physical symptoms after neurotoxic exposure. J Occup Med 30:684–686, 1988.
21. Brodsky CM: Multiple chemical sensitivities and other environmental illnesses: A psychiatrist's view. Occup Med 2:695–704, 1987.
22. Broughton A, Thrasher JD: Antibodies and altered cell-mediated immunity in formaldehyde-exposed humans. Common Toxicol, 2:155–174, 1988.
23. California Medical Association Scientific Board Task Force on Clinical Ecology: Clinical ecology: A critical appraisal. West J Med 144:239–245, 1986.
24. Council on Scientific Affairs, American Medical Association: Clinical ecology. JAMA 268:3465–3467, 1992.
25. Cullen MR: Multiple chemical sensitivities: Development of public policy in the face of scientific uncertainty. New Solutions Fall:16–24, 1991.
26. Dager SR, Holland JP, Cowley DS, Dunner DL: Panic disorder precipitated by exposure to organic solvents in the workplace. Am J Psychiatry 144:1056–1058, 1987.
27. Dalton P: Odor perception and beliefs about risks. Chem Senses 21:447-458, 1996.
28. Dalton P: Cognitive influences on health symptoms from acute chemical exposure. Health Psychol 18(6):1–12, 1999.
29. Deyo RA: The messenger under attack— Intimidation of researchers by special-interest groups. N Engl J Med 336(16):1176–1179, 1997.
30. Doty R, Deems DA, Frye RE, et al: Olfactory sensitivity, nasal resistance, and autonomic function in patients with multiple chemical sensitivies. Arch Otolaryngol Head Neck Surg 114:1422–1427, 1988.
31. Fiedler N, Kipen H: Chemical sensitivity: The scientific literature. Environ Health Perspect 103(Suppl2):409-415, 1997.
32. Gilbert ME: Neurotoxicants and limbic kindling. In Isaacson RL, Jensen KF (eds): The Vulnerable Brain and Environmental Risks. Vol. 1. Malnutrition and Hazard Assessment. New York, Plenum Press, 1992.
33. Gots RE: Multiple chemical sensitivities—public policy. Clin Toxicol 33(2):111–113, 1995.
34. Gots RE: Multiple chemical sensitivities: Distinguishing between psychogenic and toxicodynamic. Reg Toxicol Pharmacol 24(1):S8–S15, 1996,
35. Graveling RA, Pilkington A, George JPK, et al: A review of multiple chemical sensitivity. Occup Environ Med 56(2):73–85, 1999.
36. Hu H, Johnson K: A report to the State of Washington Department of Labor and Industries: A comparison of single photon emission computed tomography in normal controls, in subjects with multiple chemical sensitivity syndrome, and in subjects with chronic fatigue syndrome. Olympia, WA, Washington Department of Labor and Industries, 1999.
37. Hummel T, et al.: A double-blind, randomized, controlled investigation of olfactory and trigeminal chemoreception in healthy controls and patients with multiple chemical sensitivities, before and after challenge with 2-propanol or room air (in preparation).
38. International Programme on Chemical Safety (UNEP-ILO-WHO), et al: Conclusions and recommendations of a workshop on multiple chemical sensitivities. Reg Toxicol Pharmacol 24:S188–189, 1996.
39. International Society of Regulatory Toxicology and Pharmacology: ISRTP Board Conclusions. Reg Toxicol Pharmacol 18:79, 1993.
40. Isenberg SA, Lehrer PM, Hochron S: The effect of suggestion and emotional arousal on pulmonary function in asthma: A review. Psychosom Med 54:192–216, 1992.
41. Leznoff A: Clinical aspects of allergic disease: Provocation challenges in patients with multiple chemical sensitivity. J Allergy Clin Immunol 99(4):438–442, 1997.
42. Leznoff A: Personal communication. 1997.
43. Lundberg JM, Lundblad L, Saria A, Anggard A: Inhibition of cigarette smoke–induced edema of the nasal mucosa by capsaicin pretreatment and a substance P antagonist. Naunyn-Schmiedeberg's Arch Pharmacol 326:181–185, 1984.

44. Madison RE, Broughton A, Thrasher JD: Immunologic biomarkers associated with an acute exposure to exothermic by-products of a urea-formaldehyde spill. Envion Health Perspect 94:219–223, 1991.
45. Margolick J: Technical Report to the State of Washington Department of Labor and Industries. Olympia, WA, 2000.
46. McClelland GH, et al: The effects or risk beliefs on property values: A case study of a hazardous waste site. Risk Anal 10:485–497, 1990.
47. McKenzie JN: The production of the so-called "rose cold" by means of an artificial rose. Am J Med Sci 91:45–47, 1996.
48. Meggs WJ, Cleveland CH: Rhinolaryngoscopic examination of patients with the multiple chemical sensitivity syndrome. Arch Environ Health 48:14–18, 1993.
49. Meggs WJ, Dunn KA, Bloch RM, Goodman PE, Davidoff AL: Prevalence and nature of allergy and chemical sensitivity in a general population. Arch Environ Health 51:275–282, 1996.
50. Meggs WJ, Elsheik T, Metzger WJ, et a: Nasal pathology and ultrastructure in patients with chronic airway inflammation (RADS and RUDS) following an irritant exposure. J Toxicol Clin Tox 34:383–396, 1996.
51. Meggs WJ: Hypothesis for induction and propagation of chemical sensitivity based on biopsy studies. Environ Health Perspect 105(Suppl2):473–478, 1997.
52. Pitman RK, Orr SP, Shalev AY: Once bitten, twice shy: Beyond the conditioning model of PTSD. Biol Psychiatry 33:145–146, 1993.
53. Post RM et al: Chronic cocaine administration sensitization and kindling effects. In Raskin A, Uhlenhath EH (eds): Cocaine: Clinical and Biobehavioral Aspects. New York, Oxford University Press, 1987.
54. Post RM: Transduction of psychosocial stress into the neurobiology of recurent affective disorder. Am J Psychiatry 149:999–1010, 1992.
55. Rovee CK, Harris SL, Yopp R: Olfactory thresholds and level of anxiety. Bull Psychosom Soc 2:76–78, 1973.
56. Schneider RA: Newer insights into the role and modifications of olfaction in man through clinical studies. Ann NY Acad Sci 237:217–223, 1974.
57. Shusterman D, Balmes J, Cone J: Behavioral sensitization to irritants/odorants after acute overexposure. J Occup Med 30:565–567, 1988.
58. Simon GE, Katon WJ, Sparks PJ: Allergic to life: Psychological factors in environmental illness. Am J Psychiatry 147:901–906, 1990.
59. Simon G, Daniell W, Stockbridge H, Claypoole K, Rosenstock L: Immunologic, psychological and neuropsychological factors in multiple chemical sensitivity: A controlled study. Ann Intern Med 119:97–103, 1993.
60. Society of Nuclear Medicine Brain Imaging Council: The ethical clinical practice of functional brain imaging. J Nucl Med 37(7):1256–1259, 1996.
61. Sorg BA: Proposed animal neurosensitization model for multiple chemical sensitivity in studies with formalin. Toxicology 111:135–145, 1996.
62. Sparks PJ, Simon GE, Katon WJ, et al: An outbreak of illness among aerospace workers. West J Med 153:23–33, 1990.
63. Sparks PJ, Daniell W, Black DW, et al: Multiple chemical sensitivity syndrome: A clinical perspective. I. Case definition, case definition theories of pathogenesis and research needs. J Occup Med 36(7):718–730, 1994.
64. Sparks PJ: Idiopathic environmental intolerance. In Ballantyne, Marrs, Syversen (eds): General and Applied Toxicology, 2nd ed. London, MacMillin, 1999, pp 1703–1720.
65. Stewart DE: Environmental hypersensitivity disorder, total allergy, and 20th century disease: A critical review. Can Fam Physician 33:405–409, 1987.
66. Sullivan JB, Krieger GR: Hazardous Materials Toxicology. Baltimore, Williams & Wilkins, 1992.
67. Terr AI: Clinical ecology in the workplace. J Occup Med 31:257–261, 1989.
68. Thrasher JD, Madison R, Broughton A, Gard Z: Building-related illness and antibodies to albumin conjugates of formaldehyde, toluene diisocyanate, and trimellitic anhydride. Am J Ind Med 15:187–195, 1989.
69. Vogt RD: Use of laboratory tests for immune biomarkers in environmental health studies concerned with exposure to indoor air pollutants. Environ Health Perspect 25:85–91, 1991.
70. Vojdani A, Ghoneum M, Brautbar N: Immune alteration associated with exposure to toxic chemicals. Toxicol Ind Health 8:239–253, 1992.

RICHARD KREUTZER, MD

IDIOPATHIC ENVIRONMENTAL INTOLERANCE: CASE DEFINITION ISSUES

From Environmental Health
  Investigations Branch
California Department of Health
  Services
Oakland, California

Reprint requests to:
Richard Kreutzer, MD
Environmental Health
  Investigations Branch
California Department of Health
  Services
1515 Clay St. Suite 1700
Oakland, CA 94612

Case definitions may be used for many different purposes, such as program eligibility, clinical diagnosis, clinical studies, and population-based studies or investigations. The same phenomenon may have different case definitions for different purposes. Furthermore, the case definition for a given purpose may become more specific over time as more information about the condition becomes available. This chapter is devoted to case definitions for clinical diagnosis and population-based studies, specifically for conditions that are labeled idiopathic environmental intolerance.

The condition, or collection of conditions, here described as idiopathic environmental intolerance (IEI) also have been called multiple chemical sensitivity (MCS), environmental illness (EI), 20th-century disease, chemical hypersensitivity syndrome, total allergy syndrome, universal allergy, and cerebral allergy. The term IEI is not endorsed by patient advocates and remains controversial. It was recommended at a 1996 workshop organized by the International Programme on Chemical Safety of the World Health Organization. It was preferred over the most frequently used name, multiple chemical sensitivity, because this latter term "makes an unsupported judgement on causation."[9]

CLINICAL CASE DEFINITION ISSUES

Determining if a new disease exists can be important to the clinician for differential diagnosis, treatment decisions, and targeting prevention. The process of defining a new disease is necessarily iterative.[13] Usually, a complex of signs, symptoms or other findings will be sufficiently different to merit a new diagnostic label. The more heterogeneous the presentations and potential causes across individuals, the more difficult it is to define a new disease. In most cases, the subsequent acquisition of information about an initially-defined disease may lead to greater understanding and a more specific case definition. Over time, definition criteria may shift from manifestational elements of the history and physical exam to physiologic or laboratory findings. Observations of a newly defined condition will usually be replicated by a range of practitioners drawn from a variety of sub-disciplines and locations of practice. Affected persons may tend to have something in common, such as common exposure, common susceptibilities, or common demographic characteristics.

The common elements to be found in most of the existing clinical case definitions for IEI conditions include (1) patient reports of **multiple symptoms** (2) which are attributed to exposure to **extremely low doses** of common chemicals (Table 1). Other elements of contention include the criterion for chronicity (e.g., 3 months versus 6 months), the required number of organ systems affected, the "lowness" of the exposure level, the number and type of chemical triggers, the necessity of a precipitating exposure event, and whether other conditions such as asthma or pre-existing psychological disorders should be grounds for exclusion.[3,10,12] One thing most of these case definitions have in common is that they are almost entirely qualitative, relying on patient and clinician subjective reports of distressing symptoms and attributions to environmental exposures that have never been shown to be replicable. There are no objective correlates of the condition (e.g., clinical signs or laboratory findings).[12] Theories of underlying mechanisms for the condition have been controversial.[1,7]

Theron Randolph first proposed what is here called IEI as a disease in the late 1950's and 60's.[11] He and others attributed illnesses to modern-day synthetic chemicals and the inability of humans to adapt to these exposures. At the time, medical technologies were burgeoning and medicine was becoming increasingly sub-specialized. Some practitioners and members of the public feared that medical sub-specialists were fragmenting the body and ignoring the milieu in which disease occurred. They advocated a holistic approach to medicine and were receptive to Randolph's theories, which compared the human body to a receptacle that filled up over time with chemical insults and developed disease when it reached the point of over-flowing. A school of practitioners called "clinical ecologists" was formed and in their books and articles they described a very broad range of cases that fit their theories.

Forty years later, there is little more specificity in the case definition to aid the clinician in diagnosing a patient with this disease. There are no consistent symptoms, signs, or pathological features that distinguish this disease and there remains great controversy among the broad range of sub-disciplines about the nature of this condition. Kipen et al. describe using a questionnaire to distinguish MCS (a.k.a. IEI) cases from other clinic cases on the basis of the number of chemical incitants described by the patient as eliciting aversive responses.[6] While this instrument may prove useful for discriminating MCS patients from others, it would be unwieldy and insufficiently sensitive and specific as a diagnostic tool.

Historically, clinical ecologists advocated the use of oral challenges, unblinded inhalational exposures or skin testing as provocation tests to diagnose the condition. None of these measures have been carefully tested and validated.[5] Ashford and Miller have advocated an operational case definition for IEI that can be seen as an extension of the clinical ecology approach.[2] They have proposed that a patient with IEI could be shown to have MCS under carefully controlled double-blinded conditions when, after removal from suspected offending agents, their symptoms clear

TABLE 1. Case Definitions for Idiopathic Environmental Intolerance Conditions

Ashford and Miller (1989):
The patient with multiple chemical sensitivities can be discovered by removal from the suspected offending agents and by rechallenge, after an appropriate interval under strictly controlled environmental conditions. Causality is inferred by the clearing of symptoms with removal from the offending environment, and recurrence of symptoms with specific challenge.

Association of Environmental and Occupational Clinics 1992 Workshop on Multiple Chemical Sensitivity, Working Group on Characterizing Patients:
- A change in health status identified by the patient
- Symptoms triggered regularly by multiple stimuli
- Symptoms experienced for at least 6 months
- A defined set of symptoms reported by patients
- Symptoms that occur in three or more organ systems
- Exclusion of patients with other medical conditions (psychiatric conditions are not considered exclusionary)

Bartha et al. (1999):
- The symptoms are reproducible with repeated chemical exposure.
- The condition is chronic.
- Low levels of exposure, lower than previously or commonly tolerated, result in manifestations of the syndrome.
- The symptoms improve or resolve when the incitants are removed.
- Responses occur to multiple chemically unrelated substances.
- Symptoms involve multiple organ systems.

Clinical Ecologists (definition appearing in each issue of the journal *Clinical Ecology*):
Ecologic illness is a chronic multisystem disorder, usually polysymptomatic, caused by adverse reactions to environmental incitants, modified by individual susceptibility and specific adaptation. The incitants are present in air, water, food, drugs and habitat.

Cullen (1987):
The disorder is acquired in relation to some documentable environmental exposure(s), insult(s), or illness(es). This criteria restricts attention to patients who develop symptoms for the first time after some untoward encounter with their environment and specifically excludes patients with longstanding health problems who, later, may come to attribute certain symptoms to chemical exposure.

Symptoms involve more than one organ system. This limits attention to those patients with complex symptom patterns and eliminates, for example, patients with recurrent headaches or cough triggered by diverse stimuli.

Symptoms are elicited by exposures to chemicals of diverse structural classes and toxicologic modes of action. Individuals with classic allergic reactions to specific compounds and closely related substances (e.g., isocyanates or grains) are thus not included here.

Symptoms are elicited by exposures that are demonstrable (albeit of low level). By demonstrable we mean that people other than the patient should be aware of the chemical, e.g., smell it, even if not bothered by it. This criterion excludes frankly delusional patients and those who speculate (but cannot smell or otherwise define) that chemicals "must be present" whenever they feel poorly.

Exposure that elicits symptoms must be very low, by which we mean standard deviations below "average" exposures known to cause adverse human responses. Since data on the range of "normal" responses are often unavailable, a rule of thumb would be that exposures are known to be generally lower than 1% of established threshold limit values.

No single available test of organ system function can explain symptoms. This excludes, for example, individuals whose symptoms are attributable to bronchospasm, vasospasm, seizure disorder, or any other reversible lesion that can be identified and specifically treated. Patients in whom symptoms alone can be provoked are not excluded, nor are those who may be shown to have an underlying biochemical or immunologic abnormality, unless associated reversible organ system function can also shown.

Table continued on following page

TABLE 1. Case Definitions for Idiopathic Environmental Intolerance Conditions *(Cont.)*

Levin and Byers (1987):
"The term environmental illness is used to describe an acquired disease characterized by a series of symptoms caused and/or exacerbated by exposure to environmental agents. The triggering agents include industrial and domestic chemicals, cigarette smoke, diesel fumes, and alcoholic beverages. The symptoms involve multiple organs in the neurologic, endocrine, genitourinary and immunologic systems...the only truly novel aspect of environmental illness is the realization that similar symptom complexes frequently are seen in individuals without known 'massive' exposure and the diagnosis can be made on the basis of these symptom complexes."

National Research Council (1992), Workshop on Multiple Chemical Sensitivities, Working Group on Research Protocol for Clinical Evaluation:
• Sensitivity to chemicals. By sensitivity we mean symptoms or signs related to chemical exposures at levels tolerated by the population at large that is distinct from such well recognized hypersensitivity phenomena as IgE-mediated immediate hypersensitivity reactions, contact dermatitis, and hypersensitivity pneumonitis.
• Sensitivity may be expressed as symptoms and signs in one or more organ systems.
• Symptoms and signs wax and wane with exposures.
• It is not necessary to identify a chemical exposure associated with the onset of the condition.
• Preexistent or concurrent conditions, e.g., asthma, arthritis, somatization disorder or depression, should not exclude patients from consideration.

Nethercott et al. (1992):
• The symptoms are reproducible with exposure.
• The condition is chronic.
• Low levels of exposure result in manifestations of the syndrome.
• The symptoms improve or resolve when the incitants are removed.
• Responses occur to multiple, chemically unrelated substances.

Toronto (1985), The Ad Hoc Committee on Environmental Hypersensitivity Disorders:
"Environmental hypersensitivity is a chronic (i.e., continuing for more than 3 months) multisystem disorder, usually involving symptoms of the central nervous system and at least one other system. Affected persons are frequently intolerant to some foods and they react adversely to some chemicals and to environmental agents, singly or in combination, at levels generally tolerated by the majority. Affected persons have varying degrees of morbidity, from mild discomfort to total disability. Upon physical examination, the patient is normally free from any abnormal objective findings. Although abnormalities of complement and lymphocytes have been recorded, no single laboratory tests, including serum IgE, is consistently altered. Improvement is associated with avoidance of suspected agents and symptoms recur with re-exposure."

and then return when rechallenged by the specific agents. While theoretically appealing, this operational definition is both logistically and conceptually cumbersome.[7] These procedures would require an isolation chamber that can be inhabited for sufficient periods of time, that can exclude entirely all volatile organic chemicals to satisfy the most ardent critics, and that delivers measurable low levels of odorous chemicals using widely accepted masking techniques. There must be an ability to deliver a relatively large number of exposures and sham exposures to many different chemicals with "appropriate" clearing of the chamber and the subject's body in between. This is nearly impossible to construct. Furthermore, it is nearly impossible to develop a protocol that will accommodate the varying and conflicting periods for desensitization and adaptation that are described by different advocates. The interpretation of a set of observations for a given subject would not be straightforward since there is no agreement about the number of exposures and sham exposures required to complete the testing. Nor is there agreement about the percent of correctly identified exposures and sham exposures that would warrant diagnosing the patient as "chemically sensitive". It may be possible to construct a practical-minded protocol uniquely suited for a single subject, but the utility of doing this remains unclear.

The clinician's challenge is to apply medical science in the interests of patients who are experiencing distress. While a cure is the preferred outcome, relieving symptoms and assisting the patient with adaptation, adjustment and coping may be the most feasible outcomes. The application of a label to a person's condition can have profound affects. A label familiar to the patient can be reassuring and may carry with it a set of agreeable activities required to deal with the condition. It also can validate the patient's world-view. A label exotic to the patient can offer relief to some by simply removing some of the uncertainty of having no diagnosis at all, but it can raise anxieties for others. It can also begin the process of shifting the patient's world-view to a healthier outlook and behaviors. There is a need to establish rapport with the patient and work within their belief system. However, there is a danger in validating counterproductive values and beliefs. Thus, each clinician working with a patient who attributes their condition to chemical sensitivity must carefully weigh the benefits to the patient of applying a poorly-supported case definition and label against the costs of invalidating a patient's world-view.

While a full review of treatment options is not possible here, a general approach can be recommended. A very careful history, physical exam and laboratory work-up should be conducted to rule out or treat better-defined conditions. The history also should be aimed to get a very good description of the impact of the condition on the patient's life and its prominence in the patient's self image. Clinical tools, such as Miller's Quick Environmental Exposure and Sensitivity Inventory (QEESI), are available to assist with probing these issues and documenting the patient's changing status over time. Based upon these findings, therapeutic measures can be considered.

POPULATION-BASED STUDIES/INVESTIGATIONS
CASE DEFINITION ISSUES

As described above, the absence of an agreed upon case definition for clinical purposes creates large technical and ethical difficulties for the medical practitioner. The investigator of the condition as it presents in a population has different case definition needs and challenges. IEI can be approached in two different ways: as a new disease outbreak investigation or as a careful description of the phenomenon as it presents in the population. Both types of population-based activities will be briefly described.

When an epidemic of symptoms or disease occurs, there may be a need for rapid systematic investigation to determine the cause, describe the pattern of spread, and control or eliminate the disease in the population. An **outbreak investigation paradigm** has been developed over the years.[4] It begins with developing an initial or provisional case definition and then refining this definition as additional information is gathered. In some situations, multiple case definitions may be used simultaneously. Cases in an outbreak may be classified according to the case definition as confirmed, presumptive, or suspect. They may be symptomatic or asymptomatic. Criteria for classifying cases may be clinical, laboratory or epidemiological. As the case definition becomes more specific, cases are more frequently classified as either confirmed cases or non-cases.

For example, the cause of Legionnaire's disease was totally unknown when it occurred in Philadelphia in 1976. A case was defined as a person having either a) fever and chest x-ray evidence of pneumonia, or b) a temperature of 102° F or higher and cough. An outbreak-related case was one whose onset of illness began between July 1 and August 18, 1976 and who either attended the American Legion convention between July 21 and July 24, 1976 or who had entered the Bellevue Stratford Hotel since July 1, 1976. Subsequent to the first outbreak, this case definition continued to be used until the causal agent was finally identified and a case could be more precisely defined. It became possible to define a confirmed case as a person having a four-fold or greater serologic increase in reciprocal indirect immunofluorescent titer of 128 or more to Legionella pneumophila. Presently, more sophisticated methods of identification and typing are available.

Investigators wanting to apply the outbreak paradigm to IEI have been frustrated over the years with the absence of clinical, laboratory, or epidemiological criteria with which to classify subjects. There is little agreement about subject "caseness." Symptomatic cases are potential cases solely on the basis of their subjective attribution of symptoms to chemical exposures. Furthermore, there are no criteria to categorize an asymptomatic case. As a result, to date, the outbreak paradigm approach to IEI has made little progress.

The absence of objective markers of disease does not prevent **population-based descriptive study**, which can inform the public, policy makers and clinicians about the phenomenon. Certainly, years of psychiatric epidemiology demonstrate this. Studies can be designed to examine the qualitative reports of subjects on issues of chemical sensitivity.[8] Questions for study can include:

1) What is the prevalence of reports of chemical sensitivity in the population?
2) What kind of symptoms do subjects experience? How severe are the symptoms? And are they different or similar for different perceived exposures?
3) What kind and how many chemicals are believed to trigger these symptoms? What is the time course for triggering? And how consistent is the triggering?
4) Was there a precipitating exposure event that "caused" the problem?
5) How do subjects determine that they are sensitive to chemicals?
6) Are there qualities of chemicals subjects find most aversive?
7) How has the reported chemical sensitivity affected a person's daily activities, their relationships, their social roles, and their self-image?
8) Do people who report chemical sensitivities have similarities (e.g., demographic, co-morbid conditions, psychological characteristics)?
9) How do people's experience of chemical sensitivity change over time?
10) Compared to others in the population, what do people with reported sensitivities "know" about chemicals?
11) Do reports of chemical sensitivity vary in different populations (e.g., people with different diseases, people with different cultural experiences, victims of technological disasters, war veterans)?
12) Are there laboratory correlates with some discernable group who reports chemical sensitivities?

Thus, even in the absence of a case definition, population studies can still be performed. Such careful population-based descriptive work can form the basis for further clinical research (if important associations are discovered) and guide difficult, but necessary policy deliberations that must occur even in the absence of adequate medical information.

REFERENCES

1. American Academy of Allergy, Asthma and Immunology (AAAAI) Board of Directors. Idiopathic Environmental Intolerances. J Allergy Clin Immunol 103-1 Pt1: 36–40, 1999.
2. Ashford NA, Miller CS: Chemical Sensitivity: A Report to the New Jersey State Department of Health: Dec. 1989.
3. Barta et al. Multiple Chemical Sensitivity: A 1999 Consensus. Archives of Environmental Health 54 (3):147–149, 1999.

4. CDC training module 7: Formulating Case Definitions and Identifying Cases for Analysis. US Department of Health and Human Services Public Health Service, August 1983.
5. Fung FK: Multiple chemical sensitivities (MCS): diagnostic determinations [abstract]. Annu Meet Int Soc Technol Assess Health Care, 11: Abstract No. 229, 1995.
6. Kipen HM, Hallman W, Kelly-McNeil, et. al. Measuring chemical sensitivity prevalence: A questionnaire for population studies. Am J Public Health 85:574–577, 1995.
7. Kreutzer R, Neutra R: Evaluating individuals reporting sensitivities to multiple chemicals. Final Report of the Agency for Toxic Substances and Disease Registry: June, 1996.
8. Kreutzer R, Neutra R, Lashuay N: The prevalence of people reporting sensitivity to chemicals in a population based survey. AJE 150 (1):1–12, July, 1999.
9. Lessof M: Report of Multiple Chemical Sensitivities (MCS) Workshop. Berlin, Germany, 21–23 February 1996, PCS/96.29 IPCS, Geneva Switzerland. Human and Experimental Toxicology, 16 (4):233–4, April, 1997.
10. Nethercott JR, Davidoff LL, Curbow B, Abbey H: Multiple chemical sensitivity syndrome: toward a working case definition. Archives of Environmental Health 48 (1):19–26, Jan-Feb, 1993.
11. Randolph T: Ecologic orientation in medicine. Annals of Allergy 23:7–22 Jan, 1965.
12. Sparks PJ, Daniell W, Black DW, Kipen HM, Altman LC, Simon GE, Terr AI: Multiple chemical sensitivity syndrome: a clincal perspective 1. Case definition, theories of pathogenesis, and research needs. J Occup Med 36(7):718–729, July, 1994.
13. Wegman DH, Woods NF, Bailar JC: Invited commentary on Gulf War Syndrome: how would we know a Gulf War Syndrome if we saw one? Am J Epidemiol 146, 9:709–711, 1997.

NICHOLAS D. GIARDINO, MS
PAUL M. LEHRER, PhD

BEHAVIORAL CONDITIONING AND IDIOPATHIC ENVIRONMENTAL INTOLERANCE

From Rutgers–The State University
   of New Jersey
New Brunswick, New Jersey (NDG)
   and
UMDNJ–Robert Wood Johnson
   Medical School
Piscataway, New Jersey (PML)

Reprint requests to:
Paul Lehrer, PhD
Department of Psychiatry
UMDNJ-Robert Wood Johnson
   Medical School
671 Hoes Lane
Piscataway, NJ 08854

Idiopathic environmental intolerance (IEI) is likely a complex condition involving heterogeneous etiologic and symptom-maintaining processes. Immunologic, neurologic, endocrine, behavioral, emotional, and cognitive explanations have all been put forth to explain various manifestations of IEI. Evidence exists to support at least a partial role for some of these processes in this condition. This chapter explores the role of behavioral conditioning in IEI. While at no time do we mean to suggest that behavioral conditioning can entirely "explain" IEI (indeed, we will present data to show that it cannot), we review theories and evidence that offer behavioral conditioning processes as one possible contributor to the development of this poorly understood disorder.

PRINCIPLES OF BEHAVIORAL CONDITIONING

We begin with a review of the basic principles of some common forms of behavioral conditioning, including Pavlovian conditioning, sensitization, and generalization.

Pavlovian Conditioning

Pavlovian conditioning, also called classical conditioning, occurs when a neutral stimulus is paired with a stimulus that reflexively elicits a particular response. The pairing of the two stimuli leads to the formation of a learned association between them, such that a subsequent presentation of the originally neutral stimulus alone produces a response similar to the one elicited reflexively.

In formal terms, the originally neutral stimulus is called the conditional stimulus (CS), and the original reflex-eliciting stimulus is the unconditional stimulus (UCS). The original response to the UCS is called the unconditional response (UCR), while the one produced by the CS after it becomes associated with the UCS is termed the conditional response (CR). In Pavlov's well-known experiment, the sight of food, which reflexively brings about increased salivation in the dog (the UCR), was repeatedly paired with the sound of a bell. After several pairings of the food (UCS) with the bell (CS), Pavlov's dogs would increase their rate of salivation when presented with the bell sound alone.

In addition to discrete "artificial" stimuli (e.g., tones or lights), **contextual cues** can act as powerful CSs both experimentally and in real life. That is, any number of sensory inputs that happen to occur at the same time as the UCS presentation may subsequently act as potent CSs. In animal studies, for example, simply being placed in the room in which a UCS was administered, may, by itself, elicit a strong (conditional) response similar to that caused previously by the UCS itself. Also, an early response to an agent may act as a CS for later or secondary responses. For example, mild respiratory distress may precede the onset of more serious general symptoms in a chemical or pathogen-triggered illness. Later, similar respiratory sensations experienced under more benign circumstances may serve as a CS for other symptoms experienced in the previous illness.

This type of Pavlovian conditioning, known as **interoceptive conditioning**, may be closely related to the events that occur with IEI. Here, the CS, the UCS, or both "are delivered to the mucosa of some specific viscus,"[20a] such that the viscera become the signalers or receivers of the conditional information. Interoceptive conditioning has been implicated in the etiology of some psychological disorders that show some similarity to IEI, such as panic disorder.[3] For example, a physiological sensation, such as dizziness, that had previously occurred at the onset of (i.e., been paired with) a "real" panic attack may, under completely benign circumstances, trigger subsequent attacks. Also, infusions of lactate, a chemical normally released in the body during panic attacks, reliably triggers panic attacks in those who have had previous attacks, but not in those who have not.[17] Thus, in this case, the panic attack may be a CR elicited by lactate-induced bodily sensations.

Sensitization

Sensitization refers to the process of increased sensitivity to the effects of a stimulus following an initial exposure (or exposures). Sensitization typically occurs in the period following exposure to a **noxious stimulus** (rather than a neutral or pleasurable stimulus), and is thought to have evolved to avoid or minimize injury due to re-exposure to a harmful event. Sensitization may lead to larger evoked responses to stimuli of the same, or even smaller, intensity—even when the original stimulus is not causally related to the noxious exposure. As with Pavlovian conditioning, the stimulus need only precede or coincide with the noxious event for a learned association to form. Sensitization can occur several days, or even weeks, after the initial noxious exposure.

Generalization

Generalization refers to the ability of novel (non-CS) stimuli to regularly elicit a CR, even though they have never been paired with the UCS. New stimuli may elicit a CR as long as they are perceived to be *similar* to the CS. Often, the more similar the stimulus is to the original CS, the greater its ability to produce a CR. A well-known feature of generalization is that, as time passes, stimuli that are increasingly less similar to the original CS may develop CR-generating properties. For example, a chemical odor (the sensation of which almost invariably precedes the onset of illness symptoms) may act as a CS, so that individuals may later respond negatively to similarly smelling, but nontoxic, chemical agents. As more time passes, through stimulus generalization, other similar odors may come to elicit similar symptoms.

CONDITIONING AND IEI

Many of these conditioning phenomena have been well documented in animal and human research. In addition, sensitization and Pavlovian conditioning have been reported and experimentally produced in conjunction with the administration of, or exposure to, an almost endless variety of substances, from therapeutic drugs to known industrial toxins. It is still unclear, however, to what extent, if at all, they apply to patients with IEI. Nonetheless, there are several specific characteristics of IEI that are consistent with the development of at least some portion of this disorder by conditioning processes.

First, in most patients with IEI, it is unusual to find specific untolerated compounds that do not possess **strong sensory properties** (e.g., odor). For example, odorless chemicals are rarely identified in IEI as a source of illness or symptoms. Thus, there is at least potential for such compounds to possess value as UCSs, and, subsequently, for a particular sensory property of the compound (e.g., its odor) to serve as a CS leading to symptoms similar to those experienced from a past exposure.

Second, patients with IEI exhibit **avoidance** and **increased sensitivity** to agents in a way similar to that found in other psychological avoidance paradigms, such as is seen with simple phobias. For example, when anxiety or fear becomes strongly attached to a specific stimulus, people tend to avoid that stimulus. But, while this behavior may prevent phobic episodes (if the stimulus can be forever avoided), it also may serve to *increase* one's sensitivity to the feared stimulus, or even to fear itself. This is not to say, of course, that IEI is "all in the head." Psychological processes are now known to affect symptoms in many well-established medical disorders (e.g., asthma, hypertension, diabetes, and cancer, to name but a few). Furthermore, greater sensitivity after reduced exposure to chemicals has been well documented, for example, in relation to tobacco smoke. Both nonsmokers and recently abstinent smokers show lower olfactory thresholds for certain components of tobacco smoke than do current smokers.[22]

The potential application of conditioning processes to our understanding IEI is broad. Many physiological processes, organ systems, and physical and psychological symptoms have been associated with the disorder. Similarly, many bodily and behavioral phenomena have been shown to be modifiable by simple conditioning. An exhaustive description of these would be overwhelming. Instead, we focus on a few such processes that may hold particular promise: conditional immunomodulation, taste and odor aversion, and pharmacological sensitization. We then briefly present some theories used in other areas of behavioral medicine to explain why some individuals exhibit IEI while others do not.

CONDITIONAL IMMUNOMODULATION

Immunologic mechanisms have been proposed to explain IEI, ranging from "normal" allergic reactions to toxic environmental agents, to abnormal immune responses to harmless substances. In all cases, however, immune explanations of IEI have been hampered by a lack of consistent patterns of test irregularities or reliable links between specific compounds and immune responses.

The modulation of immune function by psychological processes, such as conditioning and stress, is called **neuroimmunomodulation** or **psychoneuroimmunology**. It was first formally demonstrated in the 1920s by Metal'nikov and colleagues, who, after pairing injections of bacterial compounds with dermal stimulation, were able to evoke large immune changes by presentation of the dermal stimulation alone. Dolin, the successor to Pavlov in St. Petersburg, and his collaborators continued this work in the 1950s, reporting success in achieving CRs of both immunoenhancement and immunosuppression in many different animals, including humans. It is probably the work of Ader and Cohen in the 1970s, though, that has stimulated most of the more recent research in this area. In addition to immune changes associated with behavioral processes, a second major impact of this field of research has been to highlight behavioral changes that often are associated with changes in immune function and modulated by interactions between immune, endocrine, and nervous systems.

Numerous studies have shown that certain immune processes can be reliably altered by pairing a neutral CS with an immunomodulatory UCS. For example, the presentation of an initially neutral signal that has been previously paired with the administration of an immune system suppressant will, on its own, lead to immunosuppression in an organism. Perhaps more interesting from a psychological and clinical perspective is the finding that the robustness of an immunomodulatory CR sometimes can be strongly affected by stress. Thus, animals that are stressed before the presentation of a CS-immunoactive UCS pairing show significant CRs to subsequent CS presentations when nonstressed animals do not.[20]

CONDITIONED ODOR AND TASTE AVERSIONS

A large body of research has provided convincing evidence that distinctive tastes and odors may serve as potent (and perhaps even prepotent) CSs, such that after even brief pairings with noxious events (e.g., pain or illness), animals—including humans—exhibit behavioral avoidance of, and negative affect and illness symptoms in response to, subsequent reexposure. Learned **taste aversions** are acquired especially quickly and easily. Only a single pairing is necessary to establish a strong association, even when a long time interval passes between exposure to the flavor and the onset of illness. This phenomenon has been well illustrated in humans in the case of food aversions following chemotherapy treatment. Without proper preventative interventions, nausea induced by chemotherapy becomes associated with food consumed before the onset of gastric symptoms. Through classical conditioning, the food (as well as similar foods and flavors via generalization) acquires CS properties and thus subsequently elicits symptoms similar to those caused by the chemotherapy. Conditional taste aversions are very sensitive. Even very small doses of toxins ingested with otherwise palatable foods lead to robust learned aversion.[21]

While somewhat less studied in humans, **odor-guided aversive conditioning** also has been demonstrated to be a robust phenomenon,[19] and may be of special interest in IEI, as the great majority of untolerated substances in patients with this disorder seem to be associated with distinct olfactory properties.[1] Odor conditioning has been explicitly suggested as an etiologic pathway to IEI by Bolla-Wilson, Wilson, and Bleecker, who presented clinical cases whose courses were consistent with classically conditioned odor aversion.[4] According to Bolla-Wilson et al., after exposure to a neurotoxic substance, the association of the odor of the substance with the symptoms of exposure lead to a conditional response whereby the odor alone will, in the future, elicit symptoms similar to that produced by the toxin itself. Through stimulus generalization, more odors over time may come to elicit similar CRs.

Recently, in a creative and well-executed series of studies, Van den Bergh and colleagues demonstrated experimentally that people may acquire physiologic and behavioral responses to odors in a way that is consistent with basic conditioning principles. In one study, for example, subjects participated in a differential conditioning paradigm in which two different odors (CSs), one with a positive valance and the other negative, were paired with the inhalation of either CO_2-enriched or normal air. Upon later testing with presentation of a CS alone, only subjects who received pairings of the foul-smelling odor with the CO_2-enriched air exhibited significant respiratory changes and somatic complaints. Those who inhaled normal air paired with either odor, or inhaled CO_2-enriched air paired with a fresh-smelling odor, showed no significant physiologic changes. This particular study has since been replicated with additional odors and types of patient populations with essentially the same result: under certain conditions, people may learn to experience physical symptoms upon reexposure to a nonharmful, but unpleasant, odor that was previously paired with a potentially noxious stimulus.

As further support for the role of Pavlovian conditioning as the mediator of this effect, one recent followup study was able to demonstrate extinction of the CR after repeated exposures to the odor CS without the CO_2 pairing (i.e., after repeated presentations of the odor alone, respiratory responses and symptoms were no longer observed).[29] While these results are not by themselves strong evidence that IEI develops according to a similar paradigm, the similarity between the hyperventilation-associated symptoms reported by subjects in these studies and those described clinically in IEI[5a] is striking.

Finally, the alarming nature of many of the physical symptoms known to accompany IEI may bring the conditioning processes full circle. That is, behavioral conditioning may not only perpetuate somatic symptoms and complaints that may have originally stemmed from a toxic exposure, but, in addition, **emotional and cognitive events** (e.g., fear, anxiety) associated with a harmful (or perceived harmful) exposure, may, through the same conditioning principles, become part of the conditional response to reexposure to environmental agents. Furthermore, these behavioral responses may themselves be accompanied by physical symptoms. Emotional responses typically include physical symptoms, such as headache, fatigue, weakness, nausea, sleep disturbance, soreness, muscle tension, chest pain, heart palpitations, breathlessness, sexual dysfunction, and concentration and memory problems.

The clinical course of IEI often is consistent with an etiologic involvement of behavioral conditioning. Shusterman, Balmes and Cone reported cases of IEI in which patients became sensitized to previously tolerated chemicals after an acute overexposure.[25] In each case, according to the authors, the odor then acted as a trigger (CS) for recurrent anxiety-associated hyperventilation symptoms, including chest pains, lightheadedness, increased perspiration, dyspnea, and resting tremors. As Shusterman et al. point out, this type of responding need not be viewed as a neurotic process, but may instead be seen as a **protective psychophysiologic response** with little or no "conscious" cognitive component. It is possible, however, that personality traits (e.g., negative affectivity) may play a greater role in the extent to which stimulus generalization occurs or to which the symptoms are seen as debilitating.[14]

Again, it is unlikely that conditioning alone is sufficient to explain reactions to environmental stimuli, such as chemicals, seen in IEI. When Staudenmayer et al. exposed patients to untolerated chemicals that were either masked by tolerated odors or presented below sensory thresholds, patients still reported symptoms.[26] The problem for conditioning explanations is not that patients reported complaints in response to odors that were below sensory threshold, as others have suggested.[2] Other interoceptive cues, such as respiratory changes or other early symptoms, are wholly capable of acting as CSs. Rather, in this double-blind, placebo-controlled study, patients' responses across trials were not consistently different for (reportedly) toxic and placebo chemicals. Thus, it is difficult to explain these results if one holds that patients' reactions are merely conditioned responses, as the unconditioned stimulus (i.e., the "toxic" agent) could not be reliably identified by patient responses.

PHARMACOLOGIC SENSITIZATION

Sensitization to pharmacologic agents by Pavlovian conditioning has been studied extensively and also may be relevant to discussions of IEI.[6] Numerous physiologic and behavioral processes have been shown to be modifiable by drug-induced conditioning. And, although the magnitude of these effects may differ depending on the drug administered and the processes affected, there is no reason to believe that conditioning cannot modify most pharmacologic effects.

Pavlovian drug conditioning occurs in much the same way and according to the same basic principles presented earlier for other types of classical conditioning. A neutral stimulus (CS) is paired with the administration of a pharmacologic agent (US), which produces a measurable physiologic or behavioral response (UCR). Subsequent to the CS-US pairings, presentation of the CS alone elicits a response (CR) related to that produced by the drug. In most cases, the post-conditioning presentation of the CS plus the drug elicits a response representing the summation of the individual effects UCR and CR,[24] showing a sensitization effect when the drug is administered in the context of its original pairing.

As with conditioned immunomodulation, **stress** may be important in determining the strength, and even direction, of pharmacologic conditioning. In one experiment, for example, Flaherty, Grigson, and Brady administered insulin to rats while they were placed either in an environment similar to or substantially different from their normal housing environment. After several days, the animals were again placed in the environment in which they had been receiving the drug, but were instead given only a saline injection. Rats who had been conditioned in a novel, and thus stressful, environment showed a hyperglycemic response to the saline, while those conditioned in the familiar environment exhibited a hypoglycemic response. The authors suggest that the release of stress hormones may act synergistically to alter the normal conditional response.

Pharmacologic sensitization and the effects of stress on conditional responses may have some application to understanding chemical sensitivities and responses in IEI. For example, conditional responses to contextual stimuli associated with exposure to physioactive or psychoactive chemicals may lead to augmented responses to subsequent exposures. This type of increased sensitivity has been reported in some IEI patients.[31] In addition, the demonstration that stress occurring at the time of conditioning may alter the conditional response to subsequent exposure to contextual stimuli associated with an exposure, may help explain the failure to document consistent responses to chemicals in persons with IEI. The **synergistic actions** of stress-related hormones and environmental agents in conditional responses may result in a variety symptom profiles, even among those with similar chemical exposures.

INDIVIDUAL DIFFERENCES

Not all individuals respond to a particular environmental stimulus in the same way. Furthermore, a given individual may not respond to different stressful stimuli with the same physiological response pattern. The former is known as **individual response specificity** (IRS), and the latter, **situational response specificity** (SRS). The potential role of these psychophysiological concepts in understanding IEI has been discussed in more detail elsewhere[16a]; however, we touch on them briefly here to help explain why, given similar environmental exposures, some individuals experience symptoms while others do not, as well as why large interindividual differences in physiological profiles and responses are seen among those who do respond to certain stimuli with somatic symptoms. Implicit in this discussion, of course, is that individual response tendencies may determine symptom profiles that become subject to conditioning processes as described above.

It has been proposed that, in some individuals, stereotypic physiological responses may **predispose** a person to psychosomatic disease.[7] For example, some individuals may respond to environmental challenge (e.g., a stressful task or exposure to a specific chemical) primarily with increased heart rate or blood pressure, while others may exhibit bronchconstriction under the same circumstances. Still others may develop a skin rash or headache. According to some conceptualizations of IRS, the first group may be at greater risk for the development of hypertension and cardiovascular disease, while the second may be more prone to chronic pulmonary disorders, such as asthma. In the case of hypertension, laboratory investigations have demonstrated that individuals at risk for hypertension (e.g., siblings of hypertensive parents) may exhibit stronger cardiovascular responses to experimental stressors than those without risk.[16] In addition, compared with control subjects, hypertensives more frequently show IRS with a maximal response from blood pressure.[8,9,11] Similarly, there is some evidence that those with asthma react to a variety of stressful stimuli with bronchoconstriction,[13] while headache patients may show tension in facial and shoulder muscles.[18,30]

According to SRS theories, different types of environmental challenges may elicit fairly **specific physiological response patterns**, depending on the particular characteristics of the challenge. For example, stressors that elicit active coping may be more likely to produce physiologic responses patterns characterized by beta-sympathetic activation, including increased heart rate and blood pressure and increased ventilation. Events that elicit more passive coping, on the other hand, may be more likely to be associated with increased alpha-sympathetic and cardiac parasympathetic activation, including peripheral vasoconstriction, decreased heart rate variability and bronchoconstriction in some individuals. Thus, in addition to any individual differences in physiologic response tendencies (i.e., IRS), a person's appraisal and coping response also may affect what type of physiologic response accompanies a stressful event. For example, if exposure is believed to be harmful and unavoidable, then a passive coping response profile might be expected: feeling faint, respiratory distress, and perhaps cardiac dysfunction. If the person perceives the exposure as harmful but escapable, then we might expect to observe a very different physiologic response, characterized instead by increased heart rate and ventilation. Those who do not assess the exposure as harmful, on the other hand, may show no physiologic arousal at all.

IMPLICATIONS FOR THE TREATMENT OF IEI

If Pavlovian conditioning phenomena are involved in the development or maintenance of IEI, then certain well-established behavioral therapies may be useful in its treatment. **Desensitization through exposure** is one such technique that holds promise for those suffering from IEI. Though this procedure may seem somewhat paradoxical to some, and stands in stark contradiction to the popular views promulgated by clinical ecologists who recommend strict avoidance of untolerated compounds, intentional exposure has proved to be an extremely effective treatment technique for behavioral problems that appear to be quite similar to IEI in many respects.

At the heart of exposure therapies is the process of *extinction*. Extinction can be thought of as an unlearning of the associations made during Pavlovian conditioning. More accurately, however, extinction probably involves the learning of new associations that override those previously made. Thus, if CS-UCS pairings lead a person to associate two stimuli and thus respond to the latter in a way similar to the reflexive response to the former (i.e., the organism learns that the CS will coincide with delivery of the UCS), then repeated presentation of the CS alone should eventually lead to a new association. The CS no longer coincides with the UCS, so the person ceases to respond to the CS with the CR. Indeed, this is what typically occurs.

Other procedures may be used to assist or enhance the therapeutic effects of exposure-based therapy. In *systematic desensitization*, for example, relaxation responses are taught to help counter the unpleasant effects brought about by exposure to the symptom-evoking stimuli. In cases where extensive stimulus generalization may make it difficult to implement desensitization, cognitive therapies, which attempt to restructure more general or elaborated responses to environmental agents that are perceived by the patient to be harmful, may be necessary or more appropriate. Consistent with trends in the treatment of many behavioral problems, there is preliminary evidence that a combination of behavioral and cognitive techniques may be helpful to those with IEI.[4,12]

Therapies informed by the conditioning processes described thus far may hold promise in the treatment of IEI; however, there are some difficulties. While exposure-based treatments have been highly successful in treating certain problems that appear to share some characteristics with IEI, such as phobias and panic disorder, other related disorders have proven to be more recalcitrant. In post-traumatic stress disorder (PTSD), for example, the vivid recall of a traumatic experience and avoidance of associated stimuli often are more resistant to behavioral extinction techniques. **Memories** for these intensely fearful events are likely to comprise **strong emotional components**. Thus, through conditioning and generalization, they may create increasingly complex and persistent networks that are easily triggered and difficult to control. There is some evidence that the extreme nature of the trauma often associated with PTSD may lead to more dramatic and perseverative neurobiologic changes in the brain that may contribute to this chronic and difficult clinical presentation.[5] In addition, stress-induced neuronal damage to brain regions involved in the formation of new memories may further impede psychological treatment attempts that rely on new learning.[23]

Patients with IEI usually do not meet criteria for PTSD. Nonetheless, chemical and psychological stress, as well as the elaboration of memory processes by conditioning, generalization, and emotional activation, may contribute to the intractability of IEI. This is not to say that conditioning-based behavioral treatment approaches should not be used. Rather, as with many disorders, it may be necessary to incorporate ancillary behavioral and pharmacological components into a comprehensive treatment program.

Finally, although a thorough treatment of the topic is beyond the scope of this chapter, **operant conditioning processes** also may contribute to, and complicate, the presentation of IEI. In operant conditioning, the frequency of an action is either increased or decreased contingent upon the type of reinforcement it produces. While perhaps less obvious than with Pavlovian conditioning, operant processes may have strong effects on patient behavior in many illnesses, including IEI. So-called sick behaviors, for example, may be subtly, or not so subtly, reinforced by the solicitous actions of family members or other significant persons in the patient's environment.[15] Dysfunctional family dynamics, or difficulties and home or at work, also can affect symptom presentation. In such cases, more comprehensive psychotherapy may be advised as an adjunct to treatment.

SUMMARY
• Several conditioning-related phenomena, including pharmacologic sensitization, conditioned immunomodulation, and odor and taste aversions, appear to share some common features with IEI and, thus, may have some application to the of understanding this enigmatic condition.

• Individual response specificity and situational response specificity are two possible explanations for individual differences observed in specific responses to environmental stimuli. The first may help explain why not all people respond the same way to the same events, and the latter provides a framework for understanding why, within the same person, different physiologic response patterns may emerge in response to different types of stressful stimuli.

• Research on conditioning-related phenomena similar to IEI may help devise treatments for this poorly understood disorder. However, there are likely to be complexities in the presentation of IEI that necessitate more comprehensive treatment approaches, incorporating other behavioral and nonbehavioral treatment strategies.

REFERENCES
1. Amundsen MA, Hanson NP, Bruce BK, et al: Odor aversion of multiple chemical sensitivities: Recommendation for a name change and description of successful behavioral medicine treatment. Regul Toxicol Pharmacol 1996;24:S116–S118.
2. Ashford NA, Miller CS: Chemical Exposures: Low Levels and High Stakes, 2nd ed. New York, Van Nostrand Reinhold, 1998.
3. Barlow DH: Anxiety and Its Disorders: The Nature and Treatment of Anxiety and Panic. New York, Guilford, 1988.
4. Bolla-Wilson K, Wilson R, Bleeker ML: Conditioning of physical symptoms after neurotoxic exposure. J Occup Med 1988;30:684–686.
5. Charney DS, Deutch AY, Krystal JH, et al: Psychobiologic mechanisms of posttraumatic stress disorder. Arch Gen Psychiatry 1993;50:295–305.
5a. Cullen MR: The worker with multiple chemical sensitivities: An overview. Occup Med 1987; 2:655–661.
6. Cunningham CL: Pavlovian drug conditioning. In van Hearen F (ed): Methods of Behavioral Pharmacology. Amsterdam, Elsevier, 1993, pp349–378.
7. Engle BT, Moos RH: The generality of specificity. Arch Gen Psychiatry 1967;16:574-581.
8. Engle BT, Bickford AF: Response specificity: Stimulus-response and individual-response specificity in essential hypertensives. Arch Gen Psychiatrt 1961;5:478–489.
9. Fahrenberg J, Foerster F, Wilmers F: Is elevated blood pressure level associated with higher cardiovascular responsiveness in laboratory tasks and with response specificity? Psychophysiology 1995;32:81–91.
10. Flaherty CF, Grigson PS, Brady A: Relative novelty of conditioning context influences directionality of glycemic conditioning. J Exp Psychol Anim Behav Process 1987;13:144–149.
11. Fredrikson M, Danielssons T, Engel BT, et al: Autonomic nervous system function and essential hypertension: Individual response specificity with and without beta-adrenergic blockade. Psychophysiology 1985;22:167–174.
12. Guglielmi RS, Cox DJ, Spyker DA: Behavioral treatment of phobic avoidance in multiple chemical sensitivity. J Behav Ther Exp Psychiatry 1994;25:197–209.

13. Isenberg SA, Lehrer PM, Hochron S: The effects of suggestion and emotional arousal on pulmonary function in asthma: A review and a hypothesis regarding vagal mediation. Psychosom Med 1992;54:192–216.

14. Kellner R: Hypochondriasis and somatization. JAMA 1987;258:2718–2722.

15. Kerns RD: Families and chronic illness. Ann Behav Med 1994;16:107–108.

16. Krantz DS, Manuck SB: Acute psychophysiologic reactivity and risk of cardiovascular disease: a review and methodologic critique. Psychol Bull 1984;96:435–464.

16a. Lehrer PM: Psychophysiological hypotheses regarding multiple chemical sensitivity syndrome. Environ Health Perspect 1997;105:479–483.

17. Liebowitz MR, Gorman J, Fyer A, et al: Biological accompaniments of lactate-induced panic. Psychopharmacol Bull 1984;20:43–44.

18. Malmo RB, Shagass C: Physiologic study of symptom mechanisms in psychiatric patients under stress. Psychosom Med 1949;11:25–29.

19. Otto T, Cousens G, Rajewski K: Odor-guided fear conditioning in rats: 1. Acquisition, retention, and latent inhibition. Behav Neurosci 1997;111:1257-1264.

20. Peeke HVS, Dark K, Ellman G, et al: Prior stress and behaviorally conditioned histamine release. Physiol Behav 1987;39:89–93.

20a. Razran G: The observable and the inferable conscious in current Soviet psychophysiology: Interoceptive conditioining, semantic conditioning, and the orienting reflex. Psychol Rev 1961;68:81–147.

21. Riley AL, Tuck DL: Conditioned taste aversions: A behavioral index of toxicity. In Braveman NS, Bronstein P (eds): Experimental Assessment and Clinical Applications of Conditioned Food Aversions. New York, Annals of the New York Academy of Sciences, 1985, pp 272–292.

22. Rosenblatt MR, Olmstead RE, Iwamoto-Schaapp PN, Jarvik ME: Olfactory thresholds for nicotine and menthol in smokers (abstinent and nonabstinent) and nonsmokers. Physiol Behav 1998;65:575–579.

23. Sapolsky RM, Uno H, Rebert CS, Finch CE: Hippocampal damage associated with prolonged glucocorticoid exposure in primates. J Neurosci 1990;10:2897–2902.

24. Schwartz KS, Cunningham CL: Tolerance and sensitization to the heart-rate effects of morphine. Pharmacol Biochem Behav 1988;31:561–566.

25. Shusterman D, Balmes J, Cone J: Behavioral sensitization to irritants/odorants after acute overexposure. J Occup Med 1988;30:565–567.

26. Staudenmayer H, Selner JC, Buhr MP: Double-blind provocation chamber challenges in 20 patients presenting with "Multiple Chemical Sensitivity." Regul Toxicol Pharmacol 1993;18:44–53.

27. Van den Bergh O, Kempynck PJ, van de Woestijne KP, et al: Respiratory learning and somatic complaints: A conditioning approach using CO2-enriched air inhalation. Behav Res Ther 1995;33:517–527.

28. Van den Bergh O, Stegen K, Van de Woestijne KP: Learning to have psychosomatic complaints: Conditioning of respiratory behavior and somatic complaints in psychosomatic patients. Psychosom Med 1997;59:13–23.

29. Van den Bergh O, Stegan K, Van Diest I, et al: Acquisition and extinction of somatic symptoms in response to odours: A pavlovian paradigm relevant to multiple chemical sensitivity. Occup Environ Med 1999;56:295–301.

30. Wittrock DA: The comparison of individuals with tension-type headache and headache-free controls on frontal EMG levels: A meta-analysis. Headache 1997;37:424–432.

ARTHUR LEZNOFF, MD, FRCPC
KAREN E. BINKLEY, MD, FRCPC

IDIOPATHIC ENVIRONMENTAL INTOLERANCES: RESULTS OF CHALLENGE STUDIES

From the Division of Clinical
  Immunology and Allergy
University of Toronto
Toronto, Canada

Reprint requests to:
Arthur Leznoff, MD, FRCPC
Division of Clinical Immunology
  and Allergy
St. Michael's Hospital and
  University of Toronto
38 Shutter St., Room 215
Toronto, Canada M5B 1A6

Psychogenic mechanisms best describe the phenomenon of idiopathic environmental intolerances.[2,5,22,23,24,26] The symptoms experienced by those affected, the short time interval between exposure and symptom onset, and the wide variety and very low dose of identified triggers are consistent with a psychogenic, rather than an allergic or toxic etiology. Challenge studies, both with known panicogenic agents and self identified triggers are strongly supportive of the concept that IEI symptoms are generated by psychophysiologic mechanisms, and are the focus of this review.

CHALLENGES WITH PANICOGENIC SUBSTANCES

Symptoms reported by patients with IEI that are characteristic of panic attacks include shortness of breath, palpitations, chest pain or discomfort, choking or smothering sensation, dizziness, vertigo or unsteady feelings, feelings of unreality, paresthesia, hot and cold flashes, sweating, faintness, trembling or shaking, and fear of dying, going crazy, or doing something uncontrolled.[6]

The diagnoses of panic attack and panic disorder are made on clinical grounds. Panic *attacks* are episodes characterized by the above-mentioned symptoms. Panic *disorder* consists of three elements: episodic panic attacks, anticipatory anxiety about panic symptoms, and phobic avoidance of triggers or situations associated with previous panic attacks.[6] Various agents or panicogenic stimuli (including intravenous sodium lactate and

35% carbon dioxide inhalation) can reproduce panic attacks in panic patients,[7,15,16,27] but are used primarily in research, not clinical settings.

In addition to having many of the characteristic symptoms of panic attack, IEI patients often exhibit both anticipatory anxiety about exposure to perceived triggers (most frequently, chemical odors), and phobic avoidance of these same triggers, thereby fulfilling all three major features of panic disorder. It is possible, therefore—at least in some patients—that IEI may represent a manifestation or variant of panic disorder rather simply a comorbid, but separate, condition.

Challenges with Intravenous Sodium Lactate Infusion

Support that IEI may be a form of panic disorder comes from studies using panicogenic stimuli. In a pilot study, five patients with self-reported IEI and typical symptoms were given intravenous sodium lactate or saline placebo infusion.[3] The individuals attributed their symptoms to "chemicals" in their environment, and had gone to considerable lengths to avoid exposure. All experienced symptoms with olfactory stimuli; one also had tactile triggers. The patients had no evidence of IgE-mediated allergy, as evidenced by negative skin tests to a panel of aeroallergens, and asthma as a cause of dyspnea was excluded by negative methacholine challenge in each case. Patients having a prior diagnosis of panic disorder or taking psychotropic medications were not included. A panel of standardized psychiatric questionnaires (Mini Structured Clinical Interview for DSM III-R, the Symptom Checklist-58, the Beck Depression Inventory, and the Hamilton Anxiety Rating Scale) was administered at baseline. Infusions were carried out in a single blind fashion first with normal saline and then with 0.5 mol/l sodium lactate. Response was assessed by the Acute Panic Inventory and a Visual Analog Scale at 10-minute intervals during the procedure. Patients were assessed by an attending psychiatrist as to whether or not DSM III-R criteria for panic were clinically present at any time.

All five individuals met DSM-III-R criteria for panic attack during sodium lactate, but not placebo infusion (Tables 1 and 2). Four of the five patients were diagnosed with panic disorder (comorbid with other anxiety and/or depressive disorders) on standardized psychiatric questionnaires. In all five patients, independent psychiatric assessment confirmed the diagnosis of panic disorder on the basis of DSM III-R criteria. Although the sample size was small, these results are those expected if IEI is in fact a variant of panic disorder in these patients.

TABLE 1. Patient Demographics and Baseline Assessment

Patient No.	Age	Gender	Diagnosis (Mini SCID)	SCL-58	BDI	HARS
1	43	F	PD	80*	1	10[†]
2	43	M	PD, SP, ETOH	66*	1	0
3	40	M		83*	3	9[†]
4	29	F	PD, DD, GAD, MDD, SP	168*	19[#]	40[†]
5	57	F	PD, SP, DD, GAD, MDD	150*	37[#]	34[†]

* Suggests significant baseline emotional disturbance.
[†] Suggests significant baseline anxiety symptoms.
[#] Suggests significant baseline depressive symptoms.
SCL 58 = Symptom Checklist-58; BDI = Beck Depression Inventory; HARS = Hamilton Anxiety Rating Scale
PD = panic disorder; ETOH = alcohol abuse; DD = dysthymic disorder; GAD = generalized anxiety disorder; MDD = major depression disorder, SP = social phobia.
From Binkley K, Kutcher S: Panic response to sodium lactate infusion in patients with multiple chemical sensitivity. J Allergy Clin Immunol 99:570–574, 1997; with permission.

TABLE 2. Patient Self-Report Response and Observer-Rated Panic Attack Incidence to Normal Saline (Placebo) and Sodium Lactate Infusion

| Patient No. | VAS of Anxiety Symptoms | | | API | | | Observer-Rated Panic Attack With | | | |
| | | | | | | | Normal Saline Infusion | | Lactate Infusion | |
	Baseline	Placebo	Lactate	Baseline	Placebo	Lactate	No	Yes	No	Yes
1	1	1	8	2	5	43	X			X
2	0	0	0	0	1	7	X			X
3	1	1	4	0	0	25	X			X
4	3	3	7	12	11	21	X			X
5	5	0	6	10	5	44	X			X

VAS = visual analog scale, API = acute panic inventory
From Binkley K, Kutcher S: Panic response to sodium lactate infusion in patients with multiple chemical sensitivity syndrome. J Allergy Clin Immunol 99:570–574, 1997; with permission.

Challenges with Single-Breath Inhalation of 35% Carbon Dioxide

A larger study examined the responses of IEI patients and control subjects to single-breath inhalation of carbon dioxide, another panicogenic stimulus.[17] Subjects fulfilled criteria for IEI as outlined previously[22] and had (1) duration of illness of at least 3 months, (2) symptoms reported in at least three organ systems, including the central nervous system, and (3) reported sensitivity to at least four substances. Diagnostic and self-report measures included the Structured Clinical Interview for DSM-IV (SCID-IV), the Health and Demographics Questionnaire, Depression Anxiety Stress Scales, Panic Frequency Questionnaire, Agoraphobic Cognitions Questionnaire, Mobility Inventory for Agoraphobia, and the Anxiety Sensitivity Index, completed at baseline. Response to challenge was assessed using the Diagnostic Symptom Questionnaire and the Subjective Units of Discomfort Scale, as well as DSM-IV criteria for panic. Inhalations were carried out in a single-blind fashion. Subjects first inhaled compressed air, and the procedure was then repeated with 35% carbon dioxide in 65% oxygen. The inhalation was considered valid if the subject inhaled at least 80% of his/her vital capacity or fulfilled DSM-IV criteria for panic attack before completing the inhalation.

Thirty-one IEI patients and 31 healthy controls completed the study. None of the subjects had any previously diagnosed psychiatric disorder. Twenty-two of 31 (71%) IEI subjects fulfilled DSM-IV panic attack criteria after CO2 inhalation, compared to 8 of 31 (26%) control subjects (p < 0.001, Fisher's Exact Test).

IEI subjects scored significantly higher than controls on self-report measures of anxiety sensitivity and panic history. The increase in panic symptoms and number of catastrophic thoughts after CO2 compared to air was greater for IEI subjects than controls, despite comparable physiological responses. The authors note that the response to CO2 suggested a tendency to over-report and possibly catastrophically misinterpret physical symptoms among IEI patients, a consistent finding among patients with panic disorder.

Fourteen of 21 (67%) IEI subjects who completed the SCID-IV fulfilled criteria for one or more mood or anxiety disorders, including specific phobia (n = 4), social phobia (3), panic disorder (2), post-traumatic stress disorder (1), generalized anxiety disorder (2), major depressive disorder (2), undifferentiated somatoform disorder (3), and past major depressive disorder (6).

As in the previous study, these results are those that would be expected if IEI was in fact a variation of panic disorder. The authors concluded that panic disorder likely accounted for at least some of the IEI symptomatology. This study extends the work on panicogenic challenges to a larger group of IEI patients and includes control subjects. It provides strong evidence that at least some patients with IEI have a neurobiological diathesis similar, if not identical, to that of panic disorder.

CHALLENGES WITH IDENTIFIED INHALATIONAL TRIGGERS

Open Inhalational Challenges with Physiological and Anatomical Assessments

Leznoff[10] noted that one of the characteristic symptom patterns of many IEI subjects (Type I), included breathlessness (without pulmonary disease), lightheadedness, confusion, weakness, palpitations, and incoordination. The other constellation (Type II), was characterized by throat symptoms, often described as "throat closing or throat swelling" (with no objective confirmation) or loss of voice. Fourteen patients with

Type I symptoms were challenged with self-identified triggers in concentrations described as definitely causing their typical symptoms. A fifteenth, who described symptoms from odorless Albuterol, was challenged with saline in a blinded experiment. End tidal or arterial pC02 was measured during or immediately after the challenges. Eleven patients, including the subject challenged with saline, in whom symptoms were reproduced, demonstrated hyperventilation with reduction in pCO2 levels (Tables 3 and 4). Symptoms included observed panic, confusion, incoordination, lightheadedness, and breathlessness. The four subjects whose symptoms were not reproduced did not hyperventilate. The only two who were treated by rebreathing into a paper bag improved rapidly despite the persistence of the trigger odor in the room. Pulmonary function studies before and after the studies were unchanged.

In these 11 patients, reported symptoms were typical of those due to hyperventilation,[2,12] although other physiological consequences of panic, anxiety, or other psychological reactions also may have been involved. These results are most compatible with a psychogenic etiology for IEI, with anxiety-induced hyperventilation and hypocarbia responsible for at least some of the symptoms.

Another study tested five IEI patients with throat symptoms as well as other typical IEI complaints (Table 5).[9] The subjects were challenged with their self-identified trigger odors with a fiberoptic laryngoscope in place just above the larynx. Phonograms were performed before and after the challenge. In four cases, no abnormalities were noted in the throat or on phonography. The fifth patient, who had reported that many scents induced hoarseness and other symptoms, was found to have vocal cord polyps. "Chemical sensitivity" disappeared when the polyps

TABLE 3. Patient Characteristics and Challenge Results

Case No.	Gender/ Age	Challenge Substance	Symptoms Before	Major Symptoms After	Duration of Challenge (min)
1	M35	Asphalt fumes*	Normal	Triad[†] & panic	3
2	F49	Disinfectant smell*	Anxiety	Triad & palpations	2
3	M53	Telephone directory	Anxiety	Triad & panic	4
4	F29	Nail polish remover	Normal	Triad & panic	5
5	F37	Hair spray	Normal	Triad & crying	5
6	F44	Disinfectant	Normal	Triad & weakness	5
7	F49	Flour (tactile)	Normal	Triad and panic	2
8	M53	New carpet	Normal	Triad & nausea	10
9	F46	Nebulized saline	Normal	Triad & retching	2
10	F54	Cigarette smoke	Hoarseness	Triad & weakness	6
11	F49	Perfume	Anxiety	Triad & weakness	6
12	F41	Perfume	Normal	Normal	15
13	M51	Bathtub sealant	Normal	Normal	15
14	M33	Aliphatic hydrocarbon solvent	Normal	Normal	15
15	F60	Perfume	Normal	Normal	15

* Challenge occurred unintentionally, prior to testing.
† Triad = breathlessness without wheezing, lightheadedness or confusion, and incoordination
From Leznoff A: Provocative challenges in patients with multiple chemical sensitivity. J Allergy Clin Immunol 99:438–442, 1997; with permission.

TABLE 4. Blood and Alveolar Gas Analysis

Case	pCO2 Before Challenge	pCO2 After Challenge	SaO2 Before Challenge	PO2 SaO2 After Challenge
1#	—	18*	—	104*
2#	—	20*	—	92*
3	22	13	98	99
4	38	22	—	—
5	39	32	98	100
6	37	29	97	104
7	30	20	94	98
8	37	27	96	98
9†	37	—	97	—
10	35	21	97	99
11	29	20	98	99
12	35	35	99	99
13	32	30	100	100
14	37	37	98	98
15	35	33	98	98

* Arterial pCO2 and PO2 (other values by end tidal pCO2 and oximeter SaO2)
# No prechallenge data—triggers experienced just prior to study
† Patient too distressed after placebo challenge. Study aborted.
From Leznoff A: Provocative challenges in patients with multiple chemical sensitivity. J Allergy Clin Immunol 99:438–442, 1997; with permission.

were removed. The reactions to odors in these four patients were felt to be psychogenic. The fifth likely exhibited the phenomenon of "symptom attribution."

Blinded Inhalational Challenges with Identified Triggers

Staudenmayer performed blinded challenges in 20 IEI patients.[23] Trigger odor (A) in identified concentrations induced typical IEI symptoms. When the same odor in the same concentration was masked by a stronger, nonoffensive self-identified scent (B), the patients could not reliably distinguish the mixture (A+B) from the inoffensive odor alone. This suggests that awareness of the chemical—not the chemical itself—caused the symptoms. These results are compatible with a psychological etiology of IEI.

Rea et al.[19] claim that their challenge studies provide confirmation of a toxicogenic etiology of chemical sensitivity. However, analysis of their data suggests the

TABLE 5. Idiopathic Environmental Illness

Patient No.	Gender/Age	Challenge Chemical	Laryngoscopy		Phonogram After
			Before	After	
1	F27	Perfume	Normal	Normal	Normal
2	F46	NH$_4$ detergent	Normal	Normal	Normal
3	F34	Cigarette smoke	Normal	Normal	Normal
4	F29	Hair spray	Normal	Normal	Normal
5	F22	Nil	Polyps	Polyps	Unchanged

From Leznoff A: Multiple chemical sensitivity: Myth or reality? Practic Allergy Immunology 8:48–52, 1993; with permission.

opposite conclusion. They challenged 100 IEI subjects with chemicals in "ambient" concentrations. Eight challenge items were randomized and double-blinded (five "chemicals" and three placebos), and one challenge exposure, a single natural gas flame, was unblinded. Each subject received multiple challenges with each item. Although several criteria for a positive result were examined, the only "significant" index was a rise in pulse rate. Fifty patients were withdrawn from the study because they "reacted so severely."

The authors did not provide an analysis of these 50, and so did not determine whether these severe reactions occurred exclusively with chemicals. Had this been the case, it is unlikely that the data would have been omitted from the report. Consequently, it is reasonable to assume that one-third (the expected fraction) of these severe reactions were in response to placebo.

There were 300 challenges to chemicals in the other 50 subjects. Only 14 (4.67%), elicited a "positive" response (significant rise of pulse rate); 286 chemical challenges (95%) failed to elicit a positive response. Placebo did not induce a positive response in this group. Complete analysis of the data, including patients who completed the study and those who were withdrawn, shows that in the vast majority of challenges, patients failed to react to their purported triggers when they were unaware of their presence. Rather than supporting a toxicogenic etiology of IEI, this study suggests a psychogenic etiology of IEI.

CHALLENGES IN PATIENTS WITH ATYPICAL FOOD SENSITIVITIES

Patients with IEI often have atypical food allergies,[11,18] and patients with multiple atypical food sensitivities often have environmental sensitivities.[18] Ingestion of identified allergenic foods produces the same subjective symptom profile as IEI. Classic allergic symptoms are absent, and allergy skin tests are negative.[13,20] Therefore, this problem can be considered to be analogous to IEI and, in many cases, a part of this syndrome. Double-blind challenge studies on such patients have consistently and unequivocally demonstrated that, when blinded, they cannot distinguish their putative allergenic food from placebo.[13,14,20] This is consistent with a psychogenic etiology of their symptoms.

UNCONTROLLED CHALLENGES IN THE POPULATION AND TIME-DEPENDENT SENSITIZATION

The failure of toxicogenic theories to explain the phenomenon of IEI has been reviewed elsewhere.[1,24] Among theoretical models are kindling and time-dependent sensitization. These are phenomena observed in animals whereby exposure to various agents (e.g., electric shock, stress, an agent such as amphetamine, cocaine, or lidocaine) results in increasing sensitivity to these agents after a period of time.[28] If this mechanism were operative in humans, it might have relevance to symptoms generation in IEI. Similar experiments with humans would be difficult to justify on an ethical basis, but in fact, have been done inadvertently. Thousands of depressed patients have received shock treatments; millions of addicts have taken large and repeated doses of amphetamine and cocaine at various time intervals; and cardiac patients and patients undergoing procedures such as liposuction have received large and repeated doses of lidocaine. There are no reports suggestive that IEI has occurred with increased frequency in these groups. These observations and other studies[28] suggest that kindling and time-dependent sensitization, as described in animals, may not be relevant to human IEI.

OTHER EVIDENCE SUPPORTING A PSYCHOGENIC ETIOLOGY OF IEI

Agents effective in treating anxiety and panic disorder, such as selective serotonin reuptake inhibitors, and methods such as relaxation training and psychological desensitization with increasing exposure to triggers have been reported to be effective in the treatment of IEI.[4,8,21,25] Clearly, larger controlled studies need to be done to fully assess the efficacy of such approaches.

SUMMARY

Symptoms reported in IEI and panic are similar, though in some patients other psychological factors and processes may operate[24] and modify the clinical picture.

Panicogenic stimuli including intravenous sodium lactate and 35% CO2 inhalation reproduce IEI symptoms diagnostic of panic in patients with IEI, but (in the CO2 study) not in controls. These results are predicted by the hypothesis that IEI results, at least in some patients, from a similar if not identical neurobiologic diathesis as panic disorder.

Reported challenge studies with self-identified triggers in IEI patients are consistent with a psychogenic etiology of this disorder.

REFERENCES

1. American Academy of Allergy, Asthma, and Immunology: Board of Directors Position Statement: Idiopathic Environmental Intolerances. J Allergy Clin Immunol 1999; 103:26–40.
2. Bass C, Gardner WN: Respiratory and psychiatric abnormalities in chronic symptomatic hyperventilation. Br Med J 1985; 290:1387–1380.
3. Binkley KE, Kutcher S: Panic responses to sodium lactate infusion in patients with multiple chemical sensitivity syndrome. J Allergy Clin Immunol 1997; 99:570–574.
4. Binkley K, Stenn P: "Specialized" psychiatric referral: Improved outcome in patients with multiple chemical sensitivity. J Allergy Clin Immunol 1998; 101:S87.
5. Black OW, Rathe A, Goldstein RB: Measures of distress in 26 "environmentally ill" subjects. Psychosomatics 1993; 34:131–138.
6. American Psychiatric Association: Diagnostic and Statistical Manual of Mental Disorders, 4th ed. Washington DC, APA, 1994.
7. Griez EJL, Lousberg H, van den Hout MA, van der Molen GM: C02 vulnerability in panic disorder. Psychiatry Res 1987; 20:87–95.
8. Guglielmi RS, Cox DJ, Spyker DA: Behavioral treatment of phobic avoidance in multiple chemical sensitivity. J Behav Ther Exp Psychiatry 1994; 25:197–209.
9. Leznoff A: Multiple chemical sensitivity: Myth or reality? Pract Allergy Immunol 1993; 8:48–52.
10. Leznoff A: Provocative challenges in patients with multiple chemical sensitivity. J Allergy Clin Immunol 1997; 99:438–442.
11. Miller C: Chemical sensitivity: History and phenomenology. (white paper) Toxicol Ind Health 1994; 10 (4/5):253–276.
12. Margarian GS: Hyperventilation syndrome: Infrequently recognized common expressions of anxiety and stress. Medicine (Baltimore) 1982; 61:219–236.
13. Parker SL, Leznoff A, Sussman GL, et al: Characteristics of patients with food related complaints. J Allergy Clin Immunol 1988; 81:351–360.
14. Pearson DJ: Food allergy, hypersensitivity, and intolerance. J Royal Coll Physicians London 1985; 19:154–162.
15. Perna G, Battaglia M, Garberi A, et al: Carbon dioxide/oxygen challenge test in panic disorder. Psychiatry Res 1994; 52:159–171.
16. Perna G, Bertani A, Arancio C, et al: Laboratory response in patients with panic and obsessive/compulsive disorders to C02 challenges. Am J Psychiatry 1995; 152:85–89.
17. Poonai N, Antony MM, Binkley KE, et al: Carbon dioxide inhalational challenges in idiopathic environmental intolerance. J Allergy Clin Immunol 2000;105:358–363.
18. Rea WJ: Chemical hypersensitivity and the allergic response. Ear Nose Throat J 1988; 67:50–66.
19. Rea WJ, Ross GH, Johnson JR, et al: Confirmation of chemical sensitivity by means of double-blind inhalant challenges of toxic volatile chemicals. Clin. Ecology 1989; 6:113–118.

20. Rix KJB, Pearson DJ, Bentley SJ: A psychiatric study of patients with supposed food allergy. Br J Psychiatry 1984; 145:121–126.
21. Selner JC, Staudenmayer H: Neurophyschophysiologic observations in patients presenting with environmental illness. Toxicol Indust Health 1992; 8(4):145–155.
22. Simon GE, Daniell W, Stockbridge H, et al: Immunologic, psychological and neurophysiological factors in multiple chemical sensitivity: A controlled study. Ann Intern Med 1993;119:97–103.
23. Staudenmayer H, Selner JC, Buhr MF: Double-blind provocative chamber challenges in 20 patients presenting with "multiple chemical sensitivity." Regul Toxical Pharmacol 1998; 18: 44–53.
24. Staudenmayer H: Environmental illness: Myth and reality. Boca Raton, Florida, Lewis Publishers, 1999.
25. Stenn P, Binkley K: Successful outcome in a patient with chemical sensitivity: Treatment with psychological desensitization and selective serotonin reuptake inhibitor. Psychosomatics 1998; 39(6):547–550.
26. Stewart DE: Psychiatric assessment of patients with "20th Century Disease ("total allergy syndrome"). Can Med Assoc J 1985; 133:1001–1006.
27. van den Hout MA, van der Molen GM, Griez E, et al: Reduction of C02-induced anxiety in patients with panic attacks after repeated C02 exposure. Am J Psychiatry 1987;144:788–791.
28. Weiss SRB, Post RM: Caveats in the use of the kindling model of affective disorders. Toxicol Ind Health 1994; 10:421–447.

PAMELA DALTON, PhD
THOMAS HUMMEL, MD, PhD

CHEMOSENSORY FUNCTION AND RESPONSE IN IDIOPATHIC ENVIRONMENTAL INTOLERANCE

From Monell Chemical Senses
  Center
Philadelphia, PA
    and
University of Dresden
Dresden, Germany

Reprint requests to:
Pamela Dalton, PhD
Monell Chemical Senses Center
3500 Market Street
Philadelphia, PA 19104

Idiopathic Environmental Intolerance (IEI; also known as Multiple Chemical Sensitivity or MCS) is a diagnosis assigned to patients who present with symptoms that are associated with exposure to generally low-level environmental chemicals.[53,70,71] IEI patients report a diverse, diffuse constellation of symptoms, including fatigue, headache, dizziness, dysesthesia, blurred vision, memory loss, and lack of concentration.

In 1987, Cullen[12] introduced **four major criteria** for a diagnosis of IEI (MCS), which have become most widely used: (1) IEI is an acquired disorder characterized by recurrent symptoms. (2) It is referable to multiple organ systems. (3) It occurs in response to demonstrable exposure to many chemically unrelated compounds at doses far below those established in the general population to cause harmful effects. (4) No single widely accepted test of physiologic function can be shown to correlate with symptoms.[53] In the United States, the number of IEI symptomatics fulfilling Cullen's criteria has been estimated at 1% of the population.[39] However, the incidence of people reporting sensitivity to one or more environmental chemicals is quite high: approximately 30% of the general population consider themselves intolerant of chemicals.[52]

The diverse set of symptoms attributed to IEI has led, not surprisingly, to numerous hypotheses regarding IEI etiology.[60] These hypotheses include changes of the immune system, acquired neurotoxicity, and behavioral conditioning involving psychophysiologic mechanisms.[4,60,63,66] Some researchers have noted that patients with IEI resemble patients treated for various psychological conditions.[6,20,65,67] Many complaints of IEI patients are difficult to differentiate from symptoms of fibromyalgia, chronic fatigue syndrome, or posttraumatic stress disorder.[5,6,20,37,38,53] In fact, with respect to standardized measures of psychiatric and neurologic function, there is a large overlap between these patient groups. For example, Fiedler et al.[83] found that IEI patients could not be differentiated on a standard battery from patients with chronic fatigue syndrome, which is characterized by fatigue, cognitive dysfunction, fever, and lymphadenopathy.[33]

DO ODORS INITIATE IEI?

Despite this diversity of hypotheses about the etiology of IEI, one feature stands out across a wide range of reports —for many respondents, **IEI appears to be provoked by the perception of odor**. The typical agents that have been claimed to initiate the sensitization process in the IEI syndrome include solvents, pesticides, paints, diesel exhaust, cleaning fluids and a variety of fragranced products.[11,75] Frequently, it is the odor of those products that appears to trigger the symptoms experienced by IEI patients,[42] and IEI patients are likely to report that they have a heightened sensitivity to odors. Although it has been recommended that IEI patients avoid exposure to odorants,[59] there is limited evidence that fragrances directly mediate the onset of IEI symptoms. An excellent, exhaustive review of the available literature by Ross et al.[63] came to the conclusion that " . . . fragrances do not initiate IEI sensitization." Nonetheless, among IEI patients and practitioners who diagnose this condition, there is a longstanding belief in the association between odors and the onset of IEI symptoms.

The association between odors and the appearance of IEI symptoms has led to the hypothesis that the **intranasal chemoreceptive senses** are specifically involved in IEI pathophysiology.[4,10,23,34,49] Although this relationship has been cited in numerous accounts of IEI etiology, only a few studies have attempted to test this hypothesis.

Are IEI Patients More Sensitive to Odors?

Doty and coworkers[23] investigated responses to odors in 18 IEI patients and compared their results to the responses obtained from age- and gender-matched, healthy controls. They assessed odor thresholds for phenyl ethyl alcohol, a rose-like odor which produces little or no trigeminal activation,[22] and methyl ethyl ketone, a mixed trigeminal-olfactory stimulant that is commonly used in solvents.[22] Additional parameters investigated were blood pressure, heart rate, respiratory rate, and nasal resistance, using anterior rhinomanometry.

Despite the belief of all participating IEI patients that they had greater-thannormal olfactory sensitivity, no significant differences between IEI patients and controls were found for odor thresholds. Doty and his colleagues provided four major explanations for this unexpected finding: (1) IEI symptoms may be related to suprathreshold rather than threshold olfactory stimuli. (2) IEI symptoms may be due to trigeminal stimulation, rather than olfactory activation. (3) Cognitive processing of odor stimuli might be altered in IEI patients, leading to an increased response to odors. (4) The two olfactory stimuli tested were simply not representative of the wealth of odors encountered in everyday life.

A major finding of the Doty et al. study was that IEI patients evidenced ". . . significantly higher total nasal resistances on both inhalation and exhalation than did the matched normal controls . . ." They also reported a higher respiratory rate in IEI patients. Both of these outcomes were interpreted as suggesting higher autonomic reactivity among IEI patients than among controls.

Hummel and coworkers[28,29] conducted a series of studies that focused on changes in both the olfactory and trigeminal systems in IEI patients, as assessed by means of electrophysiological correlates of chemoreception. Specifically, they examined whether IEI patients responded differently after they had been exposed to either room air or 2-propanol, a common solvent in cleaning fluids, cosmetics, and pesticides.[41,64] In addition, data from this group of patients were compared to healthy controls matched for age and gender.[29]

Results from 23 self-identified IEI patients meeting the Cullen criteria[12] were compared to 23 healthy controls. Subjects participated in two experiments performed on two consecutive days. The experiments were composed of two identical sessions. During the interval between sessions subjects were exposed for 10 minutes to either room air or 2-propanol at a peri-threshold concentration. The low concentration was chosen to observe whether symptomatology would occur in the absence of strong olfactory cues. Exposure was performed in a double-blind manner, i.e., neither patient nor experimenter was aware of the stimulus condition in either session. Since the concentration of 2-propanol was at the level of olfactory threshold, there was no definitive olfactory clue during exposure.

During each session, intranasal chemosensory function was assessed by means of (1) psychophysical tests for phenyl ethyl alcohol odor thresholds and odor discrimination for eight triplets of odorants, and (2) EEG-derived chemosensory event-related potentials (ERP) in response to olfactory (hydrogen sulfide, H2S) and trigeminal stimuli (carbon dioxide, CO2). Mucosal congestion was monitored using acoustic rhinometry. In addition, subjects performed an odor identification task before entering the study. Symptoms were noted verbatim according to the patient's complaint.

This study provided the following major results:

- Approximately 30% of patients diagnosed with IEI presented symptoms regardless of the type of challenge (Table 1). In contrast, only 10% of healthy controls exhibited symptoms in response to the challenge with either room air or 2-propanol. This finding suggested a relatively higher susceptibility of IEI patients to nonspecific experimental manipulations when compared with healthy controls.
- IEI patients exhibited a reduced sensitivity for suprathreshold olfactory stimuli. This was observed for both psychophysical (odor identification and odor discrimination tasks; Fig. 1) and electrophysiological measures (olfactory ERP amplitudes P1N1; Fig. 2). In addition, trigeminal ERP amplitudes were found to be significantly smaller in IEI patients.
- Consistent with previous studies,[23] IEI patients had olfactory thresholds that were not significantly different from those of healthy controls.

TABLE 1.   Symptoms Reported by Individuals Following Exposure
to Either 2-Propanol or Room Air

Exposure to 2-Propanol	Exposure to Room Air
IEI Patients	
Drowsiness, chest discomfort, stomach upset	Intranasal burning
Trembling, flushing, crying	Tiredness
Urge to sneeze	Headache
Headache	Sore throat
Sore throat, hoarseness	
Controls	
Nasal burning	Vertigo

Odor discrimination
triple forced choice; controls ■ IEI patients ☐

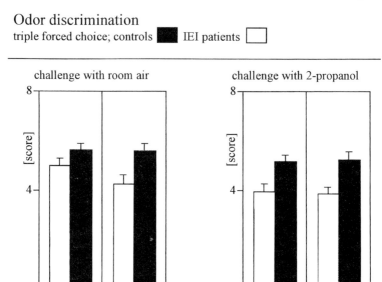

FIGURE 1. Scores for odor discrimination (means, standard errors of means) before and after challenge with either room air or 2-propanol, respectively. Olfactory discrimination is expressed as the number of correctly identified items (out of a total of 8 items); higher numbers indicate a higher sensitivity. For odor discrimination, a significant effect of the factor "group" was observed, indicating that IEI patients had a lower sensitivity to suprathreshold olfactory stimuli. In contrast, for phenyl ethyl alcohol thresholds there was no difference between groups.

- Challenges with 2-propanol did not produce effects on chemosensory function of IEI patients that differed from challenges with room air; moreover, no differences were observed between IEI patients and controls following exposure in either condition.
- Nasal volume did not change significantly in relation to the 2-propanol challenge for either group.

The observed differences between patients and controls regarding their reactions to intranasal challenge appeared to reflect changes in the cognitive processing of suprathreshold chemosensory information rather than differences in sensitivity or in sensory processing of chemical stimuli. While the results for chemosensory sensitivity are consistent with those reported by Doty et al.,[23] the absence of effects on nasal volume among IEI patients may indicate that IEI patients do not exhibit a higher degree of autonomic reactivity than do healthy controls.

Olfactory Sensitivity in Patients with Fibromyalgia Compared to IEI Patients
The discrepancy between objective assessments of olfactory sensitivity and subjective reports of response among IEI patients is consistent with the results of a similar study of 17 fibromyalgia patients and age- and gender-matched controls.[26] As in the study reported above, olfactory sensitivity was measured in an odor identification task, an odor discrimination task, and an odor threshold task using the "Sniffin' Sticks."[27] Over a period of 4 weeks prior to the investigation, none of the

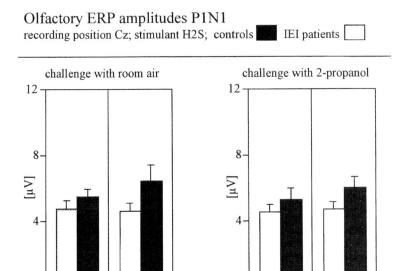

FIGURE 2. Olfactory ERP amplitudes P1N1 at recording position Cz in response to stimulation with H2S (means, standard errors of means; before and after challenge with either room air or 2-propanol). Peak amplitudes were significantly greater in controls (p = 0.014), indicating higher olfactory sensitivity compared to IEI patients.

patients took any CNS depressant drugs (e.g., tranquilizers, antidepressants, or opioids). While 65% of the patients rated their olfactory sensitivity as very high, only 33% of controls rated themselves likewise. However, when compared with controls, fibromyalgia patients had a significantly lower score for the odor identification task (p<0.05; Fig. 3). Considering the similarities between patients with fibromyalgia and IEI,[3,6,38] these data argue for **the importance of obtaining objective measures of sensitivity**. They also appear to support the findings in IEI patients of a decreased sensitivity to suprathreshold chemosensory stimuli.

In summary, when IEI patients are evaluated with objective tests of olfactory function, they appear to exhibit normal sensitivity to threshold concentrations and decreased responses to suprathreshold stimuli. In contrast, when their sensitivity to odors is assessed via self-report or other subjective measures, they appear to be more responsive and experience more adverse effects than healthy, normal control subjects. These results suggest a nonsensory locus for the distress experienced in response to chemical odors among IEI patients. This suggestion is consistent with the conclusion reached by Ross et al., after a comprehensive review of the literature on odors and IEI. Summarizing their review, Ross et al.[63] stated ". . . if IEI symptomatics have any measurable perceptual abnormality, it is in early, precognitive processing of low-level odor information . . ." This conclusion leads to the question of how much influence nonsensory (e.g., cognitive and emotional) factors can exert on chemosensory-mediated distress or adverse health symptoms. In the following text, we describe studies among non-IEI populations that examine the role of cognitive and emotional variables on people's response to chemical exposure.

Odor identification

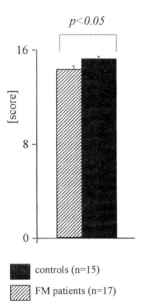

FIGURE 3. Olfactory function in 17 patients with fibromyalgia (16 female, 1 male; mean age 42 years) compared to 15 healthy controls (14 female, 1 male; mean age 45 years). Odor identification scores are expressed as the number of correctly identified items out of a total of 16 items; higher numbers indicate a higher sensitivity. Although fibromyalgia patients rated their olfactory sensitivity to be higher, they exhibited significantly lower scores for odor identification when compared to controls (p < 0.05).

ODOR SENSITIVITY AND BIAS: AN INFORMATION-PROCESSING PERSPECTIVE

Although environmental odor intolerance is a frequent complaint among IEI patients,[63] symptom reports, perceived adverse health effects and public health concerns also are increasingly precipitated by the perception of chemical odors among individuals who do not report environmental intolerance or chemical sensitivity. As a result, there has been a renewed interest in examining the mechanisms underlying the variation in the hedonic and somatic response to odors. Research has identified **two main sources of variation in olfactory response:** (1) factors that determine an individual's sensitivity to odors,[7,80,82] and (2) factors that affect the way an individual processes olfactory information.[47,73] The available evidence from studies that have compared subjective and objective olfactory responses in IEI patients and normal controls suggests that IEI patients may differ more in their processing of olfactory information than in their sensitivity to odors (see above). To help place the responses of IEI patients in the larger context of human processing of odor information, we review several lines of research that have examined the influence of cognitive, social, and attentional variables on reactions to odor among nonsensitive (normal) populations. The results from these studies have implications for interpreting the relationship between health-relevant cognitions, perceived odors, and the manifestation of environmental intolerance, particularly when related to odor and responsiveness to chemical exposure.

"Top-Down" Effects on Chemosensory Perception

It is widely acknowledged that the response to any sensory stimulus can be greatly influenced by the complex environment surrounding the exposure and the perceiver's mental state. In this view, the perception of an odor is determined by integrating the information from the volatile stimulus (e.g., "bottom-up" processing) with information that is stored in memory (e.g., "top-down" processing).[69] Bottom-up processing relies almost exclusively on the data or the information conveyed by the intensity or quality of the odor stimulus to guide perception. In contrast, top-down processing makes use of information in memory, expectations, and even the perceiver's affective or emotional state.[24,32] Remarkably, top-down processing can elicit a wide range of perceptions and responses even in the absence of any stimulus (odor) input. For instance, in a series of studies conducted by Knasko et al., exposure to a sham "malodor" (e.g., aerosolized water characterized as a malodor) led to heightened reports of discomfort and health symptoms (ranging from headaches to allergic reactions) while exposure to a sham "pleasant" odor elicited positive ratings and elevations in mood.[1,40,57]

In general, the influence of knowledge or expectation is more profound when the sensory features of a stimulus are ambiguous.[2,58] Accordingly, the propensity of odors to trigger symptom monitoring and elicit adverse symptoms may be in large part due to the ambiguous nature of many odors in everyday environments. This suggests that the heightened subjective response to odors among IEI patients may involve interactions between low-level sensory and physiological input and cognitive processes. Figure 4 illustrates the processes that can influence how an individual will interpret and respond to a chemical exposure. Within this framework, the sensory information from a volatile chemical passes through various stages of cognitive and emotional transformations. During these stages, the sensory properties of the chemical (e.g., odor intensity or quality) and the physiological effects it can produce (e.g., irritation, nasal secretions) can be influenced by cognitive and emotional factors.

Four types of nonsensory variables can influence the response to a volatile chemical in this model: (1) beliefs about the consequences of exposure to chemicals, (2) personality traits that influence the interpretation of sensations and symptoms, (3) socially-mediated cues about the effects of exposure, and (4) variation in the

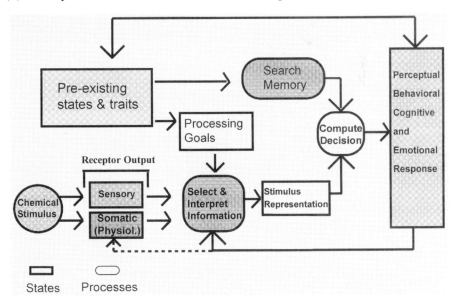

FIGURE 4. A cognitive-perceptual model of chemosensory processing, depicting the various factors and transformations that can affect an individual's interpretation and response to a volatile chemical stimulus.

focus of attention. Below, we review research that illustrates how each of these factors can influence the response to an environmental odor. The results of these studies show a number of striking parallels between the responses following laboratory studies of odor exposure in non-IEI test populations and the real-world complaints of IEI patients reporting environmental intolerances.

1. MENTAL MODELS AND CHEMOSENSORY REACTIVITY

Although symptoms and somatic sensations are based, in part, on physiological activity, they also can be influenced by general beliefs or models about illness, anatomy, and situations. For example, the degree to which we perceive ourselves to be breathless depends on our visceral respiratory sensation, but also on our understanding of any lung-related problems that we may have, knowledge of the anatomy/function of the respiratory system, the altitude at which we know ourselves to be, and the other specific contexts in which the symptoms are produced. Thus, one important source of influence on response to a chemical is the individual's accumulated knowledge or "mental model" of exposure effects. Such a schema can guide the interpretation of everyday odor experiences[61] and delimit the symptoms a person monitors and ultimately perceives.[46,50] For example, individuals living in residential areas near hazardous waste sites often report experiencing symptoms that are consistent with neurotoxic effects, even in the absence of any measurable toxic agents.[21,36,62] This outcome suggests that people can be cued to monitor and report symptoms that are related to and activated by a mental schema,[8,35,51] a mechanism that may be relevant to interpreting the odor-triggered symptom reports of IEI patients.

In a series of studies, Dalton and colleagues have examined how information about the source and consequences of exposure to a volatile chemical can meaningfully influence short-term responses to an odor stimulus.[13,14,15,19] In the basic paradigm, individuals were exposed in a chamber to a steady-state concentration of an odorant and were asked to rate the perceived intensity of odor and/or sensory irritation (i.e., eyes, nose, and throat) at regular intervals during exposure. They also completed a symptom-rating task following exposure. Although odorant concentration was held constant, subjects were told that concentration could vary or stay the same during exposure; this information minimized demand characteristics by pre-validating any change in the perceived odor intensity. In one series of studies, subjects were assigned to one of three groups that differed only with respect to the information they received from the experimenter about the odor to which they were exposed. Subjects assigned to Group Positive were told that the odorant was a natural extract distilled from a natural source. In contrast, those assigned to Group Negative were told that the odorant was an industrial chemical that has caused health problems following chronic exposures. Those assigned to Group Neutral were given no characterizing information about the odorant.

Perceived odor and irritation ratings were measured during exposure, and reports of health symptoms were obtained following exposure. In all cases, the information provided to the subject greatly influenced their experience during and following exposure to the chemical. Specifically, Dalton et al. observed that:

- The level of reported odor and irritation during exposure to acetone varied systematically with the information subjects were given about the source of the odor (Fig. 5). Subjects in Group Positive reported the lowest ratings of odor and irritation intensity during exposure, while subjects in Groups Neutral and Negative gave ratings that were significantly higher.
- Subjects in Group Negative also reported greater frequency and severity of health symptoms from exposure, including symptoms that were unassociated

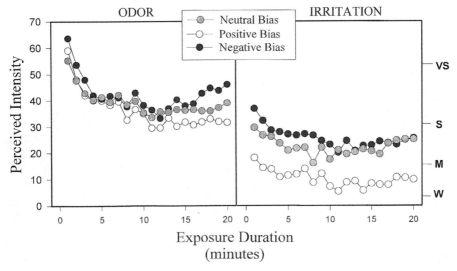

FIGURE 5.   Average intensity ratings of the perceived odor *(left panel)* and irritation *(right panel)* of 800 ppm acetone for subjects in each bias condition (n = 0/group) during a 20-minute chamber exposure to acetone. Responses given by subjects in the negative group were significantly different from those given by the subjects in the positive and the negative groups (p < .01).

with solvent exposure[30,31] and were included as a measure of response bias.[19] When exposed to a more positively evaluated odorant such as methyl salicylate (wintergreen), Groups Positive and Neutral reported significantly lower ratings of odor, irritation, and health symptoms than did Group Negative.[15]

• Subjective responses to the odor revealed differences as a function of bias group whereas objective 2-alternative, forced-choice (2-AFC), detection thresholds obtained before and after the 20-minute exposure did not. All groups showed a significant and comparable loss of sensitivity to isobornyl acetate, reflecting exposure-induced, short-term adaptation.

• The frequency of spontaneous[14] and surveyed[18,19] symptom reports varied significantly with perceived odor intensity, suggesting that symptom perception was correlated with, or perhaps triggered by, the awareness of an odor.

Interestingly, analysis of the individual participants in Group Neutral (who received no information) revealed that approximately 30% responded similarly to those given negative bias (i.e., showed little adaptation), while the rest responded similarly to those given positive bias (i.e., showed adaptation). Because bias for Group Neutral was not manipulated, these differences could be due to the subject's pre-existing models of chemical exposure, prior experience with this particular odor, or the influence of personality factors.

2. PERSONALITY TRAITS AND CHEMOSENSORY REACTIVITY

A significant amount of the variation in health and symptom perception in normal, healthy individuals can be attributed to differences in personality orientations. In general, positive affective orientations appear to lower individuals' expectancies of becoming ill, while negative orientations appear to heighten those same expectancies. **Negative affectivity** (NA)[74,77] is a personality dimension that reflects stable and pervasive differences in emotional processing, negative mood, and self-concept. Individuals who are high in negative affectivity are more likely to experience distress in the absence of overt stressors,[77] exhibit hypervigilance in scanning their environment,[74] interpret ambiguous stimuli in a negative manner,[25,77] and report more subjective health complaints.[78] These tendencies may allow environmental stimuli, such as odors, to trigger detection of baseline levels of physiological activity that would otherwise go unnoticed.[55,77–79]

Smeets and Dalton[68] conducted a study aimed at understanding the relationship between NA and responses to odor exposure. Healthy, normal volunteers who scored at the low and high extremes on the NA items of the Positive and Negative Affectivity Scale were recruited to participate. These individuals were then exposed to an odorous chemical (2-propanol) for 30 minutes, and a variety of subjective (e.g., reported symptoms) and objective (e.g., eye redness) adverse effects were measured. Before exposure, and at 5-minute intervals during exposure, subjects rated the perceived intensity of the odor and any irritation they experienced. They also rated the frequency and severity of a number of symptoms before and immediately after exposure. High NA individuals gave significantly higher ratings of irritation during exposure than did low NA individuals; following exposure, they also reported more frequent and more severe symptoms, such as eye irritation, headache, and dizziness (Figs. 6 and 7). Despite reports of high levels of eye irritation among the high NA group, no exposure-related differences in conjunctival hyperemia (redness) were observed. The heightened reports of overall irritation among the high NA individuals, coupled with their lack of concordance between subjective and objective measures of eye irritation, is consistent with the observed dissociations between objective measures of sensitivity and subjective reports to odors among individuals with IEI.

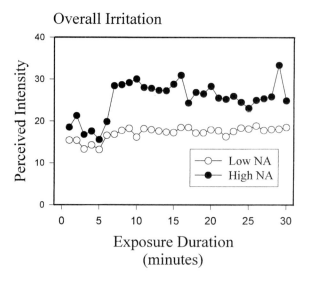

FIGURE 6.   Average intensity ratings of the perceived irritation from a 30-minute exposure to 400 ppm 2-propanol given by 24 subjects who scored high (n = 12) and low (n = 12) on the Negativity Affectivity (NA) scale. High NA individuals rated the irritation from 2-propanol exposure to be significantly more intense than low NA individuals (p <.05).

Symptom Perception

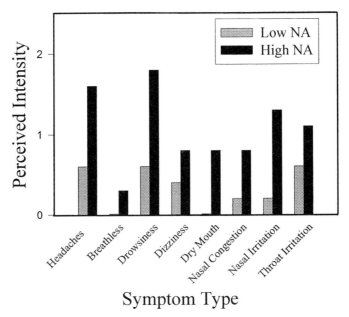

FIGURE 7. Average intensity ratings of the most frequently rated health symptoms following a 20-minute exposure to 400 ppm 2-propanol given by 24 subjects who scored high and low on the NA scale.

3. ATTENTION AND CHEMOSENSORY REACTIVITY

Exposure to volatile chemicals can elicit an array of reactions; thus, any factors that influence which signals are attended to or how the attended signals are combined and interpreted can produce enormous variation across individuals in their experience of the same sensory stimuli. Although sensory (e.g., odor, irritation) and physiological (e.g., mucus secretion) signals of exposure to a chemical often constitute a primary basis for a person's perception of exposure, these signals can be associated or dissociated from their subjective experience.[48] For example, the perception of nasal irritation can be related to physiological changes in one of three ways: (1) Complaints can occur in the absence of any increase in local inflammatory reaction; (2) Complaints can mirror genuine elevations in inflammatory response; or (3) Complaints can reflect a high baseline level that is monitored and becomes salient following some situational priming cue, such as an ambient odor. As a consequence of prior experiences or expectations, it is not unreasonable to assume that, in situations where odors are present, individuals with IEI may monitor their physiological or somatic state closely.

Dalton and Green[17] observed that strategies that alter the content of attention during exposure to a chemical can mediate the perceived magnitude of airway irritation. In those studies, subjects were asked to rate the intensity of four measures of irritation (eyes, nose, throat, and overall) at 1-minute intervals during a chamber exposure to 800 ppm acetone (a concentration that produces a strong odor, but is below the threshold for sensory irritation).[81] One-half of the subjects were given schematic diagrams of the upper respiratory airways and were asked to indicate on

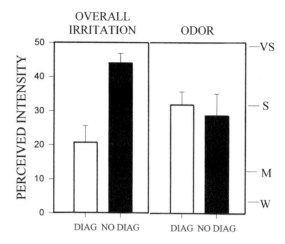

FIGURE 8.   Average intensity ratings of the perceived irritation *(left panel)* and perceived odor *(right panel)* for subjects (n = 20) who were cued to attend to the sensory aspects of exposure to 800 ppm acetone (Diagram) and for subjects (n = 20) who were not (No Diagram). The attentional manipulation had a significant effect on perceived irritation (p =.02), but not on perceived odor intensity (p > 1).

the diagram the location of the strongest nasal and/or throat irritation (e.g., stinging, burning, tingling). Other subjects rated the same measures of sensory irritation without using the diagram. Subjects who used the diagram to localize irritation, reported significantly less overall irritation than did the subjects who were not asked to localize (Fig. 8). Ratings of irritation in the nose and throat also were lower for this group. Interestingly, however, use of the diagram did not alter the rating of odor intensity or eye irritation. This suggests that focusing the subject's attention on the *concrete* sensory aspects of their experience served to reduce the overall level of irritation intensity and discomfort otherwise felt by subjects whose focus may have included both the sensory and emotional aspects of their experience. This interpretation is consistent with previous studies demonstrating that sensory monitoring during a painful experience attenuates distress, whereas attention to other aspects of the experience can amplify it.[44,45]

Everyday situations abound in which salient stimuli (such as an unexpected or unfamiliar odor) capture one's attentional focus,[54] or the situational context amplifies attention to an odor stimulus that is believed to be relevant and informative. For example, mass psychogenic illness (the collective occurrence of physical symptoms and related beliefs among one or more persons in the absence of an identifiable pathogen) often is triggered by the presence of an unfamiliar or unusual odor. This may occur because the odor stimulus orients and directs attention toward background or baseline somatic information.[9] Thus, it is possible that the attentional focus that an IEI patient deploys can determine, to a great degree, the content of their subjective experience.

4. SOCIALLY-CUED BIAS AND CHEMOSENSORY REACTIVITY

Socially mediated cues about the effects of exposure to chemicals also may play a role in the response to environmental odors among IEI patients. In a study conducted by Dalton and colleagues that employed a slight variant of the cognitive-bias paradigm, information about the consequences of exposure to a single ambient odor (acetone) was conveyed by the behavior/symptoms/verbal reports of a "confederate" subject (an actor whose positive, negative, or neutral verbalizations and symptom reports were scripted). Forty-eight subjects (16/group) were asked to rate the intensity of odor and irritation from the ambient odor during exposure. They also completed symptom questionnaires following exposure. Dalton et al.[16] found that the frequency and severity of reported irritation and "cued" symptoms were significantly higher for subjects exposed to the negative information from the confederate subject than for subjects exposed to the neutral or positive information (Figs. 9 and 10), despite the fact that no subjects reported being influenced by the comments or behaviors of the confederate subject. The individual characteristics that might predispose someone to be susceptible to this type of influence have not been articulated. However, it is possible that IEI patients may be particularly attuned to monitoring the adverse reactions of other individuals. Moreover, through increased participation in support networks, IEI patients have added exposure to reports of adverse reactions to various odorous substances, which may increase their vigilance and symptom-monitoring in the presence of odors.

Does Cognition Play a Role in Chemosensory Function and IEI?

Taken together, the results from these and other studies[40,57] provide compelling evidence that the sensory and somatic response to airborne chemical stimulation can be mediated by cognitive factors. Presuming the variation in the sensory and somatic responses of IEI patients and normal controls stemmed from differences in the cognitive processing of the signals elicited by odor exposure, at least four hypotheses can be advanced to account for the adverse symptom responses of IEI patients to environmental odors.

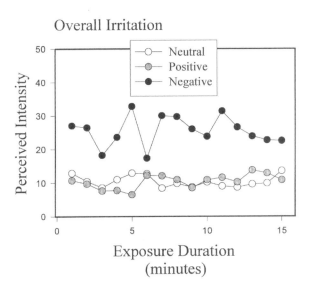

FIGURE 9. Average intensity ratings of overall irritation for 48 subjects (n = 16/group) who were exposed to 800 ppm acetone while in the presence of a confederate subject who provided either neutral, positive, or negative cues about the consequences of exposure. Subjects who were given negative cues gave significantly higher ratings of irritation than did subjects in the other two conditions (p < .05).

Symptom Perception

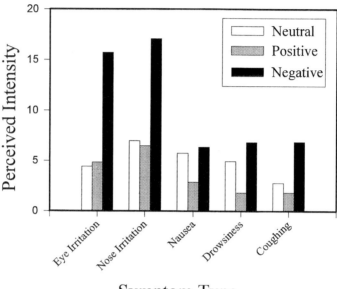

Symptom Type

FIGURE 10.   Average reported intensity for five symptoms/perceptions that were behaviorally and verbally cued by the confederate subject in the positive and negative conditions. Symptom perception differed significantly as a function of biasing condition, with subjects in the negative condition reporting higher frequency and intensity of the cued symptoms (p < .05).

First, **perceived risk** may activate or prime the retrieval from memory of a mental model of health symptoms and associated perceptions, and thus predetermine the set of symptoms or sensory systems that an individual will monitor. Previous studies and our preliminary findings suggest that people have established belief systems relating to chemical exposure effects. Thus, IEI patients may be particularly sensitive to the perceived risk of chemical exposure.

Second, the observed variation in response to odor by individuals who are high and low in negative affectivity raises the possibility that personality traits can produce difference in the **interpretations of ambiguous circumstances**. Thus, IEI patients may tend to exhibit particular personality traits that render them more susceptible to specific interpretations of their experiences.

Third, detection of an odor and the resulting concern about exposure can serve to **redirect attention** to the ambient environment and/or toward monitoring physiological and emotional status. Thus, IEI patients may be particularly prone to attend to their internal signal systems.

Finally, any or all of these mechanisms can lead to **changes in autonomic responses**, such as respiration, blood pressure, or heart rate, either as a function of the orienting response[76] or anxiety about the consequences of chemical exposure. Many researchers have raised the possibility that autonomic reactivity is elevated in IEI patients. Moreover, an awareness of heightened autonomic arousal, without explanation or correct causal attributions, can lead to spurious associations between any symptoms and a concurrently experienced odor.

CONCLUSIONS

The perception of health risks from short- or long-term exposures to volatile chemicals, frequently mediated by awareness of odors and/or irritation, is of escalating concern to the general public.[43] Moreover, research indicates that such concerns are likely to amplify the vigilance and attention paid to even low-level, neutral, background odors.[56] A common approach to addressing these health concerns has been the attempt to greatly reduce, if not eliminate, ambient concentrations of these volatiles. This approach has been used to ameliorate the symptoms of IEI patients as well. Our research suggests that interventions focused on environmental control of odors may not be an especially effective way to remediate the distress of IEI. While environmental factors certainly contribute to these (often severe and debilitating) symptoms, the findings suggest that cognitive, non-sensory factors appear to play a major role in both the initiation and maintenance of this syndrome. Just as negative information about the consequences of exposure can elevate symptom reporting, positive information about the benefits of exposure can reduce symptom reports and perceived irritation below the baseline response when no information is provided. This suggests that efforts to provide education and communication addressing the relationship between odors, irritation, perceived toxicity, and actual health risk may be of significant value for individuals who are experiencing environmental intolerances.

REFERENCES

1. Alexander RW, Fedoruk MJ: Epidemic psychogenic illness in a telephone operator's building. J Occup Med 28:42–45, 1986.
2. Anderson DB, Pennebaker JW: Pain and pleasure: Alternative interpretations for identical stimulation. Eur J Soc Psychol 10:207–212, 1980.
3. Bell IR, Baldwin CM, Schwartz GE: Illness from low levels of environmental chemicals: relevance to chronic fatigue syndrome and fibromyalgia. Am J Med 105(3A):74S-82S, 1998.
4. Bell IR, Miller CS, Schwartz GE: An olfactory-limbic model of multiple chemical sensitivity syndrome: Possible relationships to kindling and affective spectrum disorders. Biol Psychiatry 32:218–242, 1992.
5. Bell IR, Schwartz GE, Baldwin CM: Differential resting qEEG alpha patterns in women with environmental chemical intolerance, depressives and normals. Biol Psychiatry 43:376–388, 1998.
6. Buchwald D, Garrity D: Comparison of patients with chronic fatigue syndrome, fibromyalgia, and multiple chemical sensitivities. Arch Intern Med 154:2049–53, 1994
7. Cain WS, Gent JF: Olfactory sensitivity: Reliability, generality, and association with aging. J Exp Psychol Hum Percept Perform 17:382-391, 1991
8. Cavalini PM, Koeter-Kemmerling LG, Pulles MPJ: Coping with odour annoyance and odour concentrations: Three field studies. J Envir Psychol 11:123–142, 1991.
9. Colligan MJ, Murphy L: A review of mass psychogenic illness in work settings. In M. Colligan, J. Pennebaker, L .Murphy (eds): Mass Psychogenic Illness: A Social Psychological Analysis. Hillsdale, NJ, Lawrence Erlbaum, 1982.
10. Cometto-Muniz JE, Cain WS: Sensory irritation. Relation to indoor air pollution. Ann N Y Acad Sci 641:137–151, 1992.
11. Cone JE, Harrison R, Reiter R: Patients with multiple chemical sensitivities: clinical diagnostic subsets among an occupational health clinic population. Occup Med 2:721–738, 1987.
12. Cullen MR: The worker with multiple chemical sensitivities: An overview. Occup Med 2(4): 655–661, 1987.
13. Dalton P: Cognitive influences on health symptoms from acute chemical exposure. Health Psychol 18:1-12, 1999.
14. Dalton P: Odor perception and beliefs about risk. Chem Senses 21:447–458, 1996.
15. Dalton P: Cognitive influences on odor perception. Aroma-chology Review 6:2–9, 1997.
16. Dalton P, Dilks D, Ruberte J: Effects of social cues on perceived odor, irritation, and health symptoms from solvent exposure. Proceedings and Abstracts of the Annual Meeting of the Eastern Psychological Association 70:135, 1999.
17. Dalton P, Green BG: The effects of varied exposure schedule on the intensity and locus of sensory irritation from acetone. Chem Senses 21:59, 1996.

18. Dalton P, Wysocki CJ, Brody MJ, Lawley HJ: Perceived odor, irritation and health symptoms following short-term exposure to acetone. Am J Ind Med 31:558–569, 1997.
19. Dalton P, Wysocki CJ, Brody MJ, Lawley HJ: The influence of cognitive bias on the perceived odor, irritation, and health symptoms from chemical exposure. Intl Arch Occup Env Health 69:407–417, 1997.
20. Davidoff AL, Fogarty L: Psychogenic origins of multiple chemical sensitivities syndrome: a critical review of the research literature. Arch Environ Health 49:316–25, 1994.
21. Dayal HH, Baranowski T, Li Y, Morris R: Hazardous chemicals: Psychological dimensions of the health sequelae of a community exposure in Texas. J Epidemiol Community Health 48:560–568, 1994.
22. Doty RL, Brugger WE, Jurs PC, et al: Intranasal trigeminal stimulation from odorous volatiles: Psychometric responses from anosmic and normal humans. Physiol Behav 20:175–185, 1978.
23. Doty RL, Deems DA, Frye RE, et al: Olfactory sensitivity, nasal resistance, and autonomic function in patients with multiple chemical sensitivities. Arch Otolaryngol Head Neck Surg 114:1422–7, 1988.
24. Erlichman H, Bastone L: Olfaction and emotion. In Serby MJ, Chobor KL (eds): Science of Olfaction. New York, Springer-Verlag, 1992, pp 410–438.
25. Goodstein LD: Interrelationships among several measures of anxiety and hostility. J Consult Clin Psychol 18:35–39, 1954.
26. Hummel T, Cramer O, Kalden JR, Kobal G, Wendler J: Olfactory function in patients with fibromyalgia. Chem Senses 2000 (in press).
27. Hummel T, Sekinger B, Wolf SR, Pauli E, Kobal G: "Sniffin' Sticks": Olfactory performance assessed by the combined testing of odor identfication, odor discrimination, and olfactory thresholds. Chem Senses 22:39–52, 1997.
28. Hummel T, Roscher S, Jaumann JP, Kobal G: Intranasal chemoreception in patients with multiple chemical sensitivities: A double-blind investigation. Regul Toxicol Pharmacol 24:S79–S86, 1996.
29. Hummel T, Vieregge S, Roscher S, Jaumann MP, Kobal G: Double-blind comparison of intranasal chemoreception in patients with idiopathic environmental intolerances and healthy controls. (submitted) 1999.
30. Husman K: Symptoms of car painters with long-term exposure to a mixture of organic solvents. Scand J Work Environ Health 6:19–32, 1980.
31. Iregren A: Subjective and objective signs of organic solvent toxicity among occupationally exposed workers. Scand J Work Environ Health 12:469–475, 1986.
32. Isen A: Toward understanding the role of affect in cognition. In Wyer RS, Srull TK (eds): Handbook of Social Cognition. Hillsdale, NJ, Lawrence Erlbaum, 1984, pp 179–236.
33. Jason LA, Richman JA, Friedberg F, et al: Politics, science, and the emergence of a new disease. The case of chronic fatigue syndrome. Am Psychol 52:973–983, 1997.
34. Jewett DL: Research strategies for investigating multiple chemical sensitivity. Toxicol Ind Health 8:175–9, 1992.
35. Jonsson E: Annoyance reactions to environmental odors. In Turk A, Johnston Jr JW, Moulton DG (eds): Human Responses to Environmental Odors. New York, Academic Press, 1974, pp 329–333.
36. Kilburn KH, Warshaw RH: Neurotic effects from residential exposure to chemicals from an oil reprocessing facility and superfund site. Neurotoxicol Teratol 17:89–102, 1995.
37. Kilburn KH: Symptoms, syndrome, and semantics: Multiple chemical sensitivity and chronic fatigue syndrome [editorial]. Arch Environ Health 48:368–9, 1993.
38. Kipen HM, Fiedler N, Lehrer P: Multiple chemical sensitivity: A primer for pulmonologists. Clin Pulmon Med 4:76–84, 1997.
39. Kipen HM, Hallman W, Kelly-McNeil K, Fiedler N: Measuring chemical sensitivity prevalence: A questionnaire for population studies. Am J Public Health 85:574–577, 1995.
40. Knasko SC, Gilbert AN, Sabini J: Emotional state, physical well-being and performance in the presence of feigned ambient odor. J Appl Soc Psychol 20:1345–1357, 1990.
41. Koss G: Kohlenwasserstoffe. In Marquardt H, Schäfer SG (eds): Toxikologie. Mannheim, Germany, Wissenschaftsverlag, 1995, p 397.
42. Lax MB, Henneberger PK: Patients with multiple chemical sensitivities in an occupational health clinic: Presentation and follow-up. Arch Environ Health 50:425–431, 1995.
43. Lees-Haley PR, Brown RS: Biases in perception and reporting following a perceived toxic exposure. Percept Mot Skills 75:531–544, 1992.
44. Leventhal H, Brown D, Shacham S, Engquist G: Effects of preparatory information about sensations, threat of pain, and attention on cold pressor distress. J Pers Soc Psychol 37:688–714, 1979.
45. Leventhal H, Everhart D: Emotion, pain and physical illness. In Izard C (ed): Emotions in Personality and Psychopathology. New York, Plenum Press, 1979, pp 263–299.
46. Leventhal H, Meyer D, Nerenz D: The commonsense representation of illness danger. In Rachman S (ed): Medical Psychology. New York, Pergamon, 1980, pp 7–30.

47. Luce RD, Krumhansl C: Measurement, scaling and psychophysics. In Atkinson RC, Herrnstein RJ, Lindzey G, Luce RD (eds): Stevens' Handbook of Experimental Psychology. New York, Wiley & Sons, 1988, pp 137–199.
48. Mechanic D: Social psychological factors affecting the presentation of bodily complaints. New Engl J Med 82:213–225.
49. Meggs WJ: Neurogenic inflammation and sensitivity to environmental chemicals. Environ Health Perspect 101:234–238, 1993.
50. Meyer D, Leventhal H, Gutmann M: Commonsense models of illness: The example of hypertension. Health Psychol 4:115–135, 1985.
51. Miedema HME, Ham JM: Odor annoyance in residential areas. Atmos Environ 22:2501–2507, 1988.
52. Miller CS: Chemical sensitivity: Symptom, syndrome, or mechanism for disease. Toxicology 111:69–86, 1996.
53. Miller CS: White paper: Chemical sensitivity—history and phenomenology. Toxicol Ind Health 10:253–276, 1994.
54. Moray N: Attention in dichotic listening: Affective cues and the influence of instructions. Q J Exp Psychol A 11:56–60, 1959.
55. Moyle P: The role of negative affectivity in the stress process: Tests of alternative models. J Org Behav 16:647–668, 1995.
56. Neutra R, Lipscomb J, Satin K, Shusterman D: Hypotheses to explain the higher symptom rates observed around hazardous waste sites. Environ Health Perspect 94:31–35, 1991.
57. O'Mahoney M: Smell illusions and suggestion: Reports of smells contingent on tones played on radio and television. Chem Senses Flav 3:183–189, 1978.
58. Pennebaker JW: The Psychology of Physical Symptoms. New York, Springer-Verlag, 1982.
59. Randolph TG: Environmental Medicine—Beginnings and Bibliographies of Clinical Ecology. Fort Collins, Clnical Ecology Pub., 1987.
60. Rea WJ, Mitchell MJ: Chemical sensitivity and the environment. Immunol Allergy Pract 4:157–166, 1982.
61. Reiser BJ, Black JB, Abelson RP: Knowledge structures in the organization and retrieval of autobiographical memories. Cognit Psychol 17:89–137, 1985.
62. Roht LH, Vernon SW, Pier FW, Sullivan P, Ree LJ: Community exposure to hazardous waste disposal sites: Assessing reporting bias. Am J Epidemiol 122:418–433, 1985.
63. Ross PM, Whysner J, Covello VT, et al: Olfaction and symptoms in the multiple chemical sensitivities syndrome. Prev Med 28:467–480, 1999.
64. Schaller KH: 2-propanol. In Henscshler D, Lehnert G (eds): Biological Exposure Values for Occupational Toxicants and Carcinogens. Weinheim, Germany, VCH Verlag, 1994, pp 129–138.
65. Selner JC, Staudenmeyer H: Neuropsychophysiologic observations in patients presenting with environmental illness. Toxicol Ind Health 8:145–155, 1992.
66. Simon GE, Daniell W, Stockbridge H, et al: Immunologic, psychological, and neuropsychological factors in multiple chemical sensitivity. A controlled study. Ann Intern Med 119:97–103, 1993.
67. Simon GE, Katon WJ, Sparks PJ: Allergic to life: Psychological factors in environmental illness. Am J Psychiatry 147:901–6, 1990.
68. Smeets MA, Dalton P: On the influence of personality on health symptom reporting to environmental exposure. Aroma-chology Review 8:1–10, 2000.
69. Solso R: Cognitive Psychology. New York, Allyn & Bacon, 1988.
70. Sparks PJ, Daniell W, Black DW, et al: Multiple chemical sensitivity syndrome: A clinical perspective. I. Case definition, theories of pathogenesis, and research needs. J Occup Med 36:718–30, 1994.
71. Sparks PJ, Daniell W, Black DW, et al: Multiple chemical sensitivity syndrome: A clinical perspective. II. Evaluation, diagnostic testing, treatment, and social considerations. J Occup Med 36:731–737, 1994.
72. Spielman AI: Chemosensory function and dysfunction. Crit Rev Oral Biol Med 9:267–291, 1998.
73. Swets JA, Tanner WP, Birdsall TG: Decision processes in perception. Psych Rev 68:301–340, 1961.
74. Tellegen A: Structures of mood and personality and their relevance to assessing anxiety, with an emphasis on self-report. In Tuma AH, Maser JD (eds): Anxiety and the Anxiety Disorders. Hillsdale, NJ, Erlbaum, 1985, pp 681–706.
75. Terr AI: Clinical ecology in the workplace. J Occup Med 31:257–261, 1989.
76. Turpin G: Unconditioned reflexes and the autonomic nervous system. In Siddle D (ed): Orienting and Habituation. New York, Wiley & Sons, 1983, pp 1–70.
77. Watson D, Clark LA: Negative affectivity: The disposition to experience aversive emotional states. Psychol Bull 96:465–490, 1984.
78. Watson D, Pennebaker JW: Health complaints, stress, and distress: Exploring the central role of negative affectivity. Psych Rev 96:234–254, 1989.

79. Wickramasekera IE: Somatization: Concepts, data, and predictions from the high-risk model of threat perception. J Nerv Ment Dis 183:15–23, 1995.
80. Wysocki CJ, Beauchamp GK: Ability to smell androstenone is genetically determined. Proc Natl Acad Sci U S A 81:4899–4902, 1984.
81. Wysocki CJ, Dalton P, Brody MJ, Lawley HJ: Acetone odor and irritation thresholds obtained from acetone-exposed factory workers and from control (occupationally non-exposed) subjects. Am Ind Hyg Assoc J 58:704–712, 1997.
82. Wysocki CJ, Gilbert AN: National Geographic Smell Survey: Effects of age are heterogenous. In Murphy CL, Cain WS, Hegsted DM (eds): Nutrition and the Chemical Senses in Aging: Recent Advances and Current Research Needs. New York, New York Academy of Sciences, 1989, pp 12–28.
83. Fiedler N, Kipen HM, DeLuca J, et al: A controlled comparison of multiple chemical sensitivity and chronic fatigue syndrome. Psychosom Med 58:38–49, 1996.

DONALD W. BLACK, MD

THE RELATIONSHIP OF MENTAL DISORDERS AND IDIOPATHIC ENVIRONMENTAL INTOLERANCE

From the Department of Psychiatry
University of Iowa College of
  Medicine
Iowa City, Iowa

Address correspondence to:
Donald W. Black, MD
Psychiatry Research—MEB
University of Iowa College of
  Medicine
Iowa City, IA 52242-1000

The author acknowledges financial
support from the Environmental
Sensitivities Research Institute,
Baltimore, MD; the Iowa Department of Public Health; the
University of Iowa; the National
Centers for Environmental Health;
the Centers for Disease Control
and Prevention (U50/CCU711513);
and the Department of Defense
(DAMD 17-97-1)

Idiopathic environmental intolerance (IEI) is an acquired disorder with multiple symptoms, associated with diverse environmental factors tolerated by most persons, and not explained by any known medical or psychiatric disorder.[1,2,25,28] Other terms include multiple chemical sensitivity (MCS), environmental illness, and chemical hypersensitivity syndrome. IEI is not generally recognized by mainstream medicine, and a Scientific Council of the American Medical Association has urged that it not be considered a recognized diagnosis.[2] Nonetheless, a growing body of literature has documented that many persons in the United States and elsewhere have developed a similar set of symptoms, which they and some physicians attribute to an extreme sensitivity to natural and synthetic chemical "incitants."[5,11,22,30,32,38,45] Persons diagnosed with IEI are polysymptomatic, report becoming ill when exposed to low concentrations of chemicals tolerated by most people, and report that improvement is associated with avoidance of suspected compounds.[19] Most report sensitivity to multiple, unrelated compounds.[29]

THE RELATIONSHIP OF IEI TO PSYCHIATRIC DISORDERS

The diagnosis of IEI is strongly associated with psychiatric comorbidity. Though there is no particular psychiatric profile of persons with IEI, controlled[5,11,23,38] and uncontrolled studies[8,16,22,44,45,50] in which subjects have been psychiatrically assessed show a higher prevalence of mental disorder than comparison groups or to general population norms (Table 1). The conclusions of these reports

TABLE 1. Review of Twelve Case Series of Subjects with IEI in Which Psychiatric Status Is Assessed[a]

Investigator	Year	Location	# Subjects	Mean Age (range)	% Female	% With Psychiatric Symptoms/ Disorders
Brodsky[17]	1983	San Francisco	8	30 to "early 50s"	88	100
Stewart and Raskin[46]	1985	Montreal	18	38	83	100
Terr[b 45]	1986	San Francisco	50	38.5	78	—
Terr[b 46]	1989	San Francisco	90	39.5 (20-63)	70	42
Simon et al.[37]	1990	Seattle	13	—	—	92
Black et al.[11,13]	1990, 1993	Iowa City	26	49.1 (27-78)	88	87[c]
Simon et al.[38]	1993	Seattle	41	46.4	85	44[d]
Fiedler et al.[22]	1992	Piscataway	11	42 men, 43 women (28–57)	73	73
Bell et al.[5]	1995	Tucson	28	53.3	100[e]	68[f]
Witorsch et al.[50]	1995	Washington, DC	61	47.3 (27–66)	85	100[g]
Fiedler et al.[23]	1996	Piscataway	23	42	83	44
Black[8]	1996	Iowa City	4	43.7 (39–52)	50	100

[a] Different methods were used to determine psychiatric symptoms, but were counted if they yielded a definite diagnosis, or significantly abnormal ratings on self-report assessments, such as the Minnesota Multiphasic Personality Inventory.
[b] Overlapping data sets.
[c] Only 23 of 26 were assessed for psychiatric symptoms.
[d] Defined as current "panic disorder, generalized anxiety disorder, or major depression."
[e] Only women were studied.
[f] Defined as "depression, anxiety, panic."
[g] A psychiatric diagnosis was assigned in the 43 subjects assessed for DSM-III-R disorders.

have been criticized,[20] but despite their methodologic differences and wide variation in both assessment and sample selection, all relevant studies point toward the same conclusion. Depending on the assessment procedure used, the prevalence of psychiatric disorder is 42–100%. Mood, anxiety, somatoform, and personality disorders are the most frequently diagnosed conditions. Psychotic disorders are relatively uncommon and have not been linked with IEI.[10,38] Substance use disorders, which are common, also have not been linked with IEI.[5,10,38,47] While there is no clear explanation for the latter finding, it may be that the personality structure or health beliefs of someone predisposed to IEI may preclude the development of substance abuse. The next few paragraphs highlight the findings of relevant studies that address the connection between psychiatric illness and IEI.

Reports Showing the Relationship between Psychiatric Disorders and IEI

In one of the first reports from the mainstream literature, Brodsky[17] reviewed the histories of eight subjects who sought worker's compensation for injuries reportedly induced by allergic responses to substances in the workplace. The presence of allergies was not confirmed by physical examination or laboratory evidence. According to Brodsky,[14] all had a history of chronic psychiatric symptoms and were thought unable to find a place for themselves within traditional social networks.

Stewart and Raskin[44] reported on 18 "environmentally ill" persons referred to a university psychiatric consult-liaison service in Canada.[46] All were diagnosed with psychiatric disorders, including somatoform disorders (7), anxiety disorders (4), schizophrenia (3), mood disorders (3), and personality disorders (1).

Terr[45] published a case series describing the experience of 50 "environmentally ill" subjects seen in an allergy clinic in San Francisco, and later added 40 cases.[46] A review of medical records indicated premorbid psychiatric diagnoses in 38. These individuals were reported to have long, involved histories of multisystem complaints, and displayed clinical features of hypochondriasis, somatization, conversion disorder, anxiety, depression, and obsessive behavior.

Simon et al.[37] evaluated a group of 36 workers exposed to chemicals in an aerospace equipment manufacturing plant, 13 of whom were reported to develop chemical sensitivity. All but one of the latter met criteria for a psychiatric disorder, and these authors concluded that the complaints of chemical sensitivity were related to a preexisting history of psychological distress. Simon et al.[38] later evaluated 41 persons recruited from a clinical ecology practice in the Seattle area, and compared them to a control group of 34 chronic musculoskeletal pain patients. There were no differences between the groups on an extensive panel of immunologic measures or neuropsychological tests, yet they were significantly different in terms of psychiatric diagnoses. Forty-four percent of the subjects met current criteria for panic disorder, generalized anxiety disorder, or major depression, and 47% met criteria for a preexisting psychiatric condition. The figures among control subjects were 15% and 35%, respectively.

Black et al.[10] studied 26 persons diagnosed as environmentally ill by a clinical ecologist, and of 23 who consented to a psychiatric assessment using the Diagnostic Interview Schedule (DIS),[34] found that 65% met lifetime criteria for a mood, anxiety, or somatoform disorder, compared with 28% of 46 age- and gender-matched community controls. These authors also evaluated axis II disorders (reviewed later in this article) and found that when both axis I and axis II conditions were combined, only three subjects (13%) failed to meet criteria for any disorder.[10,13] They concluded that chemically sensitive patients frequently suffer from unrecognized psychological distress, which probably accounts for some or all of the symptoms attributed to environmental illness by their clinical ecologist.

Fiedler et al.[22] published the findings of 11 cases selected on the basis of Cullen's[19] definition for MCS, and reported that eight had an identifiable premorbid psychiatric condition. Fiedler et al.[23] later reported results from a controlled study of 23 subjects diagnosed with MCS. They noted that only 26% qualified for a current axis I psychiatric diagnosis, although 43% qualified for a lifetime diagnosis, most commonly depression, anxiety, or somatization. Among their normal controls, none met criteria for a current psychiatric diagnosis, and only 11% met criteria for a lifetime psychiatric diagnosis. Using the Minnesota Multiphasic Personality Inventory (MMPI),[18] subjects with IEI achieved abnormally high scores on a number of subscales, including hypochondriasis and hysteria. For example, 66% of IEI subjects met criteria for a "two point code type" (e.g., hysteria and hypochondriasis, or depression and hypochondriasis), but the figure was only 6% for controls.

Witorsch et al.[50] reported on their experience with 61 IEI patients, all but one of whom were plaintiffs in litigation. These authors found that all 43 cases in whom psychiatric assessments were made qualified for a psychiatric diagnosis. The most common diagnoses were various somatoform disorders, followed by mood disorders, personality disorders, and anxiety disorders. Only one subject had a substance-use disorder.

Bell et al.[5] evaluated 28 women diagnosed with IEI, and based on their self-reported medical history, 68% reported a past diagnosis of depression, anxiety, or panic compared to 20% of a normal comparison group.

Finally, Black et al.[8] reported four cases diagnosed with IEI who were plaintiffs in litigation. Black concluded that all met criteria for either major depression, panic disorder, or both, the symptoms of which had led a clinical ecologist to diagnose IEI. In each case, the diagnosis of IEI was felt to have been actively promoted by a clinical ecologist, leading Black to conclude that IEI can be iatrogenically produced.

The Meaning of Particular Diagnoses

The particular psychiatric disorders identified in persons diagnosed with IEI merit comment. Anxiety disorders are common, and some investigators have observed that the symptoms of IEI strongly resemble panic disorder with agoraphobia.[3,10,39] Many patients with IEI report "chemical reactions," a cluster of symptoms occur whose onset and resolution strongly suggest panic attacks; this probably explains the high frequency of panic disorder among the subjects.[10,38] The phobic avoidance many develop has been called "toxic agoraphobia," since it is functionally indistinguishable from agoraphobia.[29] Other evidence suggesting that IEI-related complaints are anxiety based comes from challenge studies and treatment case reports.[3,9,43] Leznoff[31] exposed 15 subjects to their self-reported "trigger" chemicals, which induced hyperventilation in 73% along with a rapid fall in PCO_2. Binkley and Kutcher[7] administered sodium lactate to five persons with IEI, inducing a panic attack in each. (Sodium lactate is a known panicogenic agent in persons with panic disorder.) More recently, Stenn and Binkley[43] described a case in which paroxetine and desensitization were successful in treating the panic attacks and avoidance behavior in a person "allergic" to chemicals, joining cases reported by Amundsen[3] and Black and Sparks[43] in which behavioral therapy was used to treat avoidance behavior in persons with IEI.

Other investigators have characterized IEI as a somatoform disorder.[24,36] Many persons diagnosed with IEI, in fact, appear to meet criteria for somatization disorder even before the onset of chemical sensitivity.[38] However, not all IEI patients are polysymptomatic, and many have an illness onset after age 30 years and fail to meet criteria for somatization disorder. Hypochondriasis may be an appropriate designation for many, since persons diagnosed with IEI generally are preoccupied with having an illness whose existence cannot be objectively verified.[8] Because the illness behavior is reinforced in many cases by physicians (i.e., clinical ecologists), the hypochondriasis may be iatrogenic. In some cases, a patient's belief in being chemically sensitive and having IEI attains the status of an *overvalued idea*, which is a belief maintained despite evidence to the contrary. For example, Black and Sparks[9] reported the case of a hospitalized woman diagnosed with IEI who improved with behavioral therapy, yet maintained her illness belief. Thus, even when successfully challenged, some patients do not reject the illness belief.

Some investigators[9] have compared persons diagnosed with IEI to patients with obsessive-compulsive disorder (OCD) because the former appear to have recurrent, anxiety-provoking fears and worries about chemicals and irritants, as well as behaviors (e.g., wearing a mask) that resemble compulsive rituals. Although the comparison is apt, the recurrent thoughts of most individuals diagnosed with IEI are generally not perceived as intrusive or unwanted, and are not resisted to any degree.

Persons diagnosed with IEI typically view their beliefs as rational and their behavior as appropriate, unlike persons with OCD.

Dimensional Assessment of Emotional Distress

Dimensional measures show differences between persons diagnosed with IEI and controls, and confirm that the former suffer substantial emotional distress[5,13,22,23,38] (Table 2). Relevant studies show that persons diagnosed with IEI are more likely than control subjects to have mood, anxiety, or other physical and emotional complaints, to have abnormal elevations on personality profiles, and to affirm dimensions of hypochondriasis. For example, Black et al.[13] presented findings from the Illness Behavior Questionnaire (IBQ)[33] and Symptom Checklist-90-R (SCL-90-R).[21] Data from the IBQ showed that subjects with IEI scored significantly higher than control subjects on the dimensions of disease conviction, psychological versus somatic perception of illness, and affective inhibition. *Disease conviction* refers to preoccupation with symptoms, rejection of a doctor's assurance, and affirmation that physical illness exists. *Affective inhibition* refers to difficulty in expressing feelings, especially negative ones, to others. A low score on the measure *psychological vs. somatic perception of illness* refers to a tendency to reject responsibility for one's illness and to perceive a need for medical, not psychological, treatment. The measure also indicates a tendency to somatize concerns.

TABLE 2. Summary of Dimensional Psychological Testing
in Chemically Sensitive Persons

Study	Year	# Subjects	Assessment	Findings*
Simon et al.[37]	1990	13	SCL-90-R	Elevated depression, anxiety, somatization scales
			Whiteley Index	Elevated
			BAS	Elevated
			PDQ	Elevated
Fiedler et al.[22]	1992	11	MMPI	Elevated hypochondriasis, hysteria, depression scales
Black et al.[13]	1993	22	IBQ	Elevated disease conviction, psychologic v. somatic perception of illness, affective inhibition scales
			Whiteley Index	Elevated
		21	SCL-90-R	Elevated somatization, obsessive-compulsive, depression, phobic anxiety, general severity scales
Simon et al.[38]	1993	41	SCL-90-R	Elevated depression, anxiety, somatization scales
Bell et al.[5]	1995	28	SCL-90-R	Elevated somatization, obsessive-compulsive, depression, anxiety, phobic anxiety, general severity scales
Fiedler et al.[23]	1996	18	MMPI-2	Elevated hypochondriasis, hysteria, schizophrenia, social introversion scales
			MMPI-2	Elevated anxiety, depression, health concerns, negative treatment indicators scales

* In comparison to control data or national norms
SCL-90-R = Symptom Checklist-90-Revised[21]; BAS = Barsky Amplification Scale[4]; PDQ = Personality Diagnostic Questionnaire[26]; IBQ = Illness Behavior Questionnaire[33]; MMPI = Minnesota Multiphasic Personality Inventory.[18]

On the Whiteley Index, comprised of 14 of the items from the IBQ shown to discriminate between hypochondriacal and non-hypochondriacal patients, subjects with IEI obtained relatively high scores.[33] They were more likely than control subjects to report awareness of bodily symptoms; to be bothered by many different symptoms, including aches and pains; to believe that something is seriously wrong with their bodies; to believe that their illness is not taken seriously by others; and to find it difficult to be reassured by their physicians. Black et al. concluded that persons diagnosed with IEI show a strong preoccupation with their bodily sensations and symptoms and, similar to an individual with hypochondriasis, probably amplify normal sensations. They are convinced they have a serious illness and are upset that it is not taken seriously by others. They are not easily reassured by physicians that there is nothing to worry about. Interestingly, persons diagnosed with IEI were not phobic about the illness. They denied having fears or worries about IEI.

Black et al.[13] reported that subjects with IEI received significantly higher scores than controls on the SCL-90-R for the somatization, obsessive-compulsive symptoms, depression, phobic anxiety, and general severity index scales, confirming the substantial psychological distress experienced by the subjects. These dimensional findings are partly compatible with those of Simon et al.,[38] who reported elevated scores on the Whiteley Index, and the depression, anxiety, and somatization subscales of the SCL-90-R in a sample of subjects with IEI. Bell et al.[5] also reported elevations on the depression, anxiety, somatization, obsessive-compulsive, phobic anxiety, and general severity index of the SCL-90-R for subjects with IEI, but not controls.

Personality Characteristics of Persons with IEI

Abnormal character traits are common in persons with IEI, though no particular personality profile has been identified. Black et al.[13] assessed personality disorder using the Structured Interview for DSM-III Personality Disorders (SIDP),[41] and in a sample of 23 persons with IEI found that 17 (74%) met criteria for at least one personality disorder, compared with 28% of a control group. They also met criteria for a greater number of personality disorders (1.7 vs. 0.3) and a greater number of abnormal personality traits (16.8 vs. 10.7). Of the 11 personality disorder types assessed, the schizotypal, histrionic, narcissistic, dependent, avoidant, and compulsive types were all overrepresented.

Of course, the endorsement of criteria for a personality disorder or its treatment may not have anything to do with long-standing personality traits in these individuals, but rather may be connected to the behaviors that develop in response to receiving the diagnosis. For example, IEI beliefs may be interpreted as "odd" or "magical" (schizotypal personality) or may lead to a focus on the "special nature of one's problems" (narcissistic personality), and treatment may lead to "avoiding social or occupational activities" (avoidant personality). Although the diagnosis of personality disorder implies enduring maladjustment, clinical ecologists would argue that the appearance of these traits in IEI patients represents a transient disturbance resulting from the turmoil associated with developing a serious and polysymptomatic disorder, which necessitates major changes in one's lifestyle.

Based on their personal observations, Rosenberg et al.[35] have described the personality style of many persons diagnosed with IEI as "obsessive/paranoid," which describes persons who seek medical explanations for physical symptoms and convey their history in a precise, detailed, and fastidious way. They also have described a "histrionic/somatizing" type who presents his or her history in a more global, affect-laden, and impressionistic manner. They believe the former type of patient is more difficult to work with than the latter, as they are less likely to accept psychological explanations of the disorder.

THE IOWA FOLLOW-UP STUDY OF PERSONS WITH IEI

The Iowa study began in 1988 with an intensive psychiatric assessment of 26 "environmentally ill" persons, diagnosed by a clinical ecologist, who were recruited from support groups, clinic populations, and word-of-mouth.[10,13] The study's purpose was to assess their symptoms, treatments, and attitudes towards both conventional medicine and chemical sensitivity. Black and colleagues assessed subjects for both major mental (axis I) and personality (axis II) disorders and administered questionnaires to assess mood, personality, somatic concern, and hypochondriacal behavior. The data was contrasted to that of a group of persons from the general population matched for age and gender. The subjects with IEI indicated a strong interest in their diagnosis, were mostly satisfied with their clinical ecologist, and were dissatisfied with traditional medical approaches. They reported varying treatments, including dietary restrictions, avoidance of offending agents, and physical treatments such as neutralizing injections. (The findings for axis I and II disorders and dimensional measures are reviewed earlier in this article.)

In 1997, Black et al.[15] re-interviewed 18 (69%) of the original subjects. Their mean age was 60 years, with a range from 36 to 87 years. Seven subjects refused to participate, and one could not be located (although she was still living); none had died. All still believed they were chemically sensitive, but only 7 (39%) remained under a clinical ecologist's care. All but two subjects acknowledged that their diagnosis was controversial. The subjects were using fewer treatments in 1997 than in 1988. In particular, fewer used primrose oil, charcoal/cotton filter masks, or cleansing enemas. Fifteen subjects (83%) had modified their home to make it safer. More than half (56%), reported having received treatment in a special hospital for the environmentally ill. Subjects showed a strong interest in their condition; all acknowledged reading about IEI, and 11 (62%) were currently attending support groups. All but two reported being pleased with their current IEI treatment program.

The following case report from the Iowa cohort shows the continuity of illness belief over a 9-year period.

Case report.   In 1988, Mr. A, a 29-year-old shopclerk, reported suffering a toxic brain syndrome, which made him sensitive to environmental pollutants. The disorder, he believed, began with a sensitivity to farm chemicals, but had spread to involve everything from underarm deodorant to perfume. He described symptoms such as mental confusion, speech difficulties, and even loss of consciousness.

Mr. A was well until age 26, when his sensitivities began, but was presently disabled. He had sought treatment at many hospitals, including one that specialized in treating environmental illnesses. He moved to a town in the Southwest after his physician recommended that he relocate for reasons of health. His small Iowa community banded together to help raise money for the move. Back in Iowa to visit his family, Mr. A readily agreed to an interview. He used a wheelchair, believing a sensitivity to chemicals had severely weakened his lower extremities. He felt improved living in the Southwest, and reported following a special rotation diet, taking hypoallergenic vitamins and neutralizing drops to build immunity, and using oxygen when necessary. He lived in a special trailer free of carpeting and drapes. His main treatment was avoidance of "bad" chemicals. He expressed confidence in his clinical ecologist, but not the conventional physicians who told him that his symptoms were psychologically based. He socialized mainly with other chemically sensitive persons met through a support group.

In 1997, we located Mr. A, now 36, living in his hometown, having returned from the Southwest several years earlier. He lived in a one-bedroom apartment, and, until being awarded disability benefits 2 years earlier, had been helped by his community, which had organized money to pay his living expenses. He no longer used a wheelchair, and said he had gradually regained his strength but was still careful to follow his clinical ecologist's recommendations. He rated himself as "very much improved" despite ongoing symptoms including joint pains, sore throat, and headaches, all of which he attributed to IEI. He still followed a rotation diet, took supplemental hypoallergenic vitamins, and avoided chemical exposures by restricting his social life. He had not married, nor experienced an intimate relationship. Friendly and cooperative, Mr. A displayed a bland affect and a detached, aloof manner. Clearly interested in his disorder, he conveyed a near childlike satisfaction with his special position in the community created by the illness.

In assigning a lifetime psychiatric diagnosis, we gathered raw interview data, questionnaires, and hospital records. In the past, Mr. A had received a diagnosis of an atypical conversion disorder because no medical explanation was found for his complaints of lower limb weakness. He had a remote history of major depression, and met current and lifetime criteria for an undifferentiated somatoform disorder. (He had multiple unexplained somatic complaints, but failed to meet criteria for somatization disorder.)

The Iowa follow-up showed that persons diagnosed with IEI retain their illness belief and continue to endorse symptoms that contributed to their original diagnosis even after 9 years. Without exception, these subjects continued to believe they had IEI, and continued to report multiple somatic complaints. The subjects understood the controversial nature of their disorder, but that knowledge had not undermined their confidence in the diagnosis. They remained satisfied with their medical care, though one subject complained that her mainstream doctors made her feel like a "pariah." The frequency of psychiatric diagnoses at follow-up was substantially higher than those originally reported. While the original study diagnoses were based solely on the DIS, the figures in the follow-up were based on a best-estimate method, in which all relevant data is taken into account. To illustrate: A 75-year-old woman was diagnosed in 1988 with generalized anxiety disorder (GAD) using the DIS. Now 84, her 1997 interview and medical records dating back to the 1930s confirm an episode of major depression that required treatment (diagnosed at the time as "psychoneurosis") as well as GAD. None of the subjects met current or lifetime criteria for a substance use disorder, a finding that other groups of investigators also have reported in subjects with IEI.

The prevalence of somatization disorder also was much higher than in 1988 (50% versus 17%). Several subjects missed a diagnosis of somatization disorder in 1988 by one or two symptoms, and now meet criteria. The additional time for symptoms to accumulate and to be reported by subjects, combined with less stringent DSM-IV criteria for somatization disorder (requiring 8 symptoms rather than 13), and the use of the best-estimate method probably help explain the increased prevalence. The high rate of anxiety disorder, particularly panic disorder, probably reflects the fact that for many subjects their description of chemical reactions is nearly indistinguishable from panic attacks.

All but two subjects reported feeling improved from the time of their first interview, and most subjects, on the whole, were less outwardly symptomatic. They used fewer treatments, and fewer remained under the care of a clinical ecologist than in 1988. Nonetheless, most still modified their lives to conform to the disorder. Avoidance was still a common coping device, and most continued to be less social than before developing IEI. Although five subjects (28%) indicated that they had "recovered" or "remitted," upon review of their interview and questionnaire data only two (11%) appeared to be entirely asymptomatic; that is, had no symptoms and no longer followed any treatments. And, despite the self-reported improvement, subjects remained virtually as symptomatic as when first assessed according to SCL-90-R and IBQ results. In fact, these subjects' responses to the questionnaires were not statistically different from when originally interviewed, and yet with both instruments there were substantial differences from the comparison group. SCL-90-R results show that subjects differed from the comparison sample along the obsessive-compulsive, somatization, and general symptom dimensions. This data provides further confirmation of the diagnostic data showing high rates of both somatization and anxiety disorders, and was not unexpected. The IBQ confirmed that subjects remain preoccupied with their symptoms, reject responsibility for their illness, seek medical, not psychological treatments, and remain hypochondriacal.

Family Psychiatric Disorders and IEI

Black et al.[10] found that first-degree relatives of persons diagnosed with IEI were significantly more likely than relatives of comparison subjects to have a mental disorder. Depression, alcoholism, panic disorder, and antisocial personality were more frequent, as were suicide attempts and psychiatric care (including medication/ electroconvulsive therapy, counseling, and hospitalization). These results are consistent, in part, with those of Bell et al.[6] who found high rates of alcohol and drug use disorders in the relatives of chemically sensitive persons not meeting criteria for IEI.

The meaning of an association between a family history of mental illness and IEI is unclear, but it could reflect the substantial psychiatric comorbidity found in the subjects with IEI: the subjects may simply come from families genetically "loaded" for mental disorders. The families may be similar to those described with "depression spectrum disease" (DSD) by Winokur.[49] This disorder is defined as unipolar depression occurring in persons with a first-degree relative who suffers from alcoholism or antisocial personality. In contrast to other forms of depressive illness, DSD patients are more likely female, and are more likely to develop symptoms of somatization. Personality traits typical of DSD patients include fearfulness, demanding behavior, need for reassurance and lifelong nervousness, complaining, and irritability.[47] Many of these traits also characterize individuals with IEI.

The family dynamics of persons diagnosed with IEI have not been well studied, so it is difficult to speculate on how the family of origin may have influenced the development of IEI. A report by Staudenmeyer et al.[42] found a higher prevalence of both physical and sexual abuse among a cohort of women who reported chemically related illness than in a group of control subjects with chronic medical or psychological disorders. These authors hypothesized that the etiology of the chemically related complaints may somehow be related to childhood trauma. Of course, childhood trauma in general correlates both with disturbed family dynamics and to family psychiatric illness. Thus, families of persons diagnosed with IEI may be dysfunctional simply because so many of their members suffer from mental illness. A parent with depression, alcoholism, or antisocial personality, for example, could contribute to a poor home environment as a direct result of their psychiatric illness.

PERSIAN GULF WAR VETERANS AND IEI

Chemical sensitivity has been discussed as a possible explanation for many of the complaints reported by veterans of the Persian Gulf War (PGW). Black and colleagues[14] set out to explore the association between IEI and PGW service in a sample of Iowa veterans. The study involved telephone interviews with 3695 subjects (76% of those eligible) randomly selected from one of four study domains (PGW regular military, PGW national guard/reserve, non-PGW regular military, and non-PGW national guard/reserve), stratifying for age, gender, race, rank, and branch of military service.[27]

Based on the results, Black et al.[14] reported that military personnel who participated in the PGW reported a significantly higher prevalence of symptoms of depression, post-traumatic stress disorder, chronic fatigue, cognitive dysfunction, bronchitis, asthma, fibromyalgia, alcohol abuse, anxiety, and sexual discomfort. They authors also assessed the prevalence of IEI and its risk factors. For this analysis, they developed an operational definition for IEI, which requires that a person report illness from chemical sensitivity, report sensitivity to two or more types of incitants, have symptoms in at least two organ systems, and manifest evidence of impairment or behavioral change and response to the perceived sensitivity (Table 3).

A total of 169 (3.4%) subjects met operational criteria for IEI. Among those who met criteria for IEI, more than a quarter (29%) had previously reported a physician diagnosis of IEI. Common sensitivities reported in this group included organic chemicals and solvents (83%), vehicle exhaust (69%), cosmetics (60%), pesticides/herbicides/fertilizers (48%), and cigarette smoke (48%). Prior treatments of their chemical sensitivity included lifestyle change, use of masks/gloves/special clothes, and special vitamin supplements or diet.

Military personnel deployed to the Persian Gulf were nearly twice as likely to report symptoms suggestive of IEI as the nondeployed; they also were more likely to

TABLE 3.   The Iowa Persian Gulf Study Criteria for IEI

• Routine or normal levels of exposure to chemical agents/substances (e.g., gasoline, hairspray, paint, perfume, soap) caused respondent to feel ill.

• Sensitivity (or illness following exposure) is reported to two or more of the following:

Smog/air pollution	New buildings
Cigarette smoke	Carpeting, drapery
Vehicle exhaust/fumes	Organic chemicals, solvents, glues, paints, fuel
Copiers, printers, office machines	Cosmetics, perfumes, hair spray, deodorants, nail polish
Newsprint	Other
Pesticides, herbicides, fertilizers	

• Symptoms are reported from two or more of the following categories
  Constitutional (e.g., fever, night sweats, fatigue, weight loss, weight gain)
  Rheumatologic (e.g., joint pain, muscle aches)
  Neurologic (e.g., headaches, sensory loss, tingling, paralysis)
  Cardiovascular (e.g., palpitations)
  Gastroenterologic (e.g., gas, bloating, abdominal pain)
  Dermatological (e.g., rash, blisters)
  Pulmonary (e.g., shortness of breath, cough, wheezing)
  Cognitive (e.g., confusion, difficulty concentrating, memory loss)

• Symptoms lead to a behavioral change in one or more of the following ways:
  Wearing a mask, gloves, or special clothes
  Changing one's lifestyle to minimize chemical exposure
  Moving to a new home/location
  Use of special vitamins, supplements, or diets
  Use of oxygen, antifungals, or neutralizing injections/drops

report having received a physician diagnosis of IEI, as well as sensitivity to smog, cigarette fumes, vehicle exhaust, organic chemicals and solvents, and cosmetics, perfumes, or hair spray. The deployed were more likely than the nondeployed to report changing their lifestyle in response to chemical sensitivity. Subjects meeting criteria for IEI were at increased risk for all medical and mental health conditions assessed, except for alcohol abuse and cancer. For exmaple, they had more than 10 times the odds for reporting symptoms of major depression than personnel without IEI. Multivariate logistic regression suggested several independent risk factors for IEI, including deployment to the Gulf; prior professional psychiatric treatment, and the presence of current depression, panic, or generalized anxiety disorder. Other risk variables significant at the 5% level or less are shown in Table 4.

No personality instruments were included in the interview, although several questions that tap antisocial traits were examined for their relationship to IEI. None of these items proved to have an important association with IEI. Clinical research suggests that many persons diagnosed with IEI have abnormal personality traits, but do not appear to be at risk for antisocial personality disorder. The subjects with IEI were not at risk for alcohol abuse, a finding consistent with clinical samples.

Black et al.[14] concluded that PGW veterans were almost twice as likely as non-PGW military personnel to report symptoms suggestive of IEI, and that persons with symptoms suggestive of IEI had a higher prevalence of current psychiatric symptoms and disorders. Though this cross-sectional study was not designed to assess premorbid psychiatric comorbidity, subjects were asked about prior professional psychiatric treatment and prior psychotropic medication usage (occurring before August 1990), and both variables showed a robust association with symptoms of IEI. Because a significant risk factor for IEI was a physician diagnosis of the same, it could be that iatrogenic reinforcement plays a role both in acceptance and maintenance of illness belief.

TABLE 4.   Summary of Results of Univariate Logistic Regression Analysis of Risk Factors for IEI in PGW Sample

Risk factor	Odds ratio	CI_{95}
Physician-diagnosis of IEI	27.8	15.1, 51.0
GAD, current	11.4	5.5, 22.1
Panic disorder, current	11.2	5.1, 24.9
PTSD, current	10.3	4.3, 24.8
Depression, current	8.7	5.5, 13.8
Prior professional psychiatric treatment	4.0	2.5, 6.4
Prior psychotropic drug usage	3.1	1.0, 9.5
Gender[a]	2.6	1.3, 5.2
PGW deployment[b]	1.9	1.2, 3.0
Age[c]	1.7	1.0, 2.7
Level of preparedness[d]	0.6	0.4, 0.8

GAD = generalized anxiety disorder, PTSD = Posttraumatic stress disorder, PGW = Persian Gulf War
[a] women are at greater risk than men
[b] deployed are at greater risk than nondeployed
[c] persons > 25 years are at greater risk than those < 25 years
[d] persons with low preparedness (based on sum of responses to 6 questions) are at greater risk than those with high preparedness

Health-Related Quality of Life

Black et al.[12] examined health-related quality of life in subjects meeting criteria for IEI. They were significantly more likely than the comparison group to report prolonged bed days of care (> 12 days in the past year); Veteran's Administration disability status; receiving Veteran's Administration compensation; and having a medical disability. They also were more likely to report being unemployed, and had more physician outpatient visits, emergency room visits, and inpatient hospital stays. Persons meeting criteria for IEI had lower scores on each of the 10 subscales than comparison subjects on the Medical Outcomes Survey Short form-36 (SF-36).[48] The greatest differences between the two groups were in physical role, general health, emotional role, and pain-related impairment.

These findings suggest that persons diagnosed with IEI report substantially more impairment in important domains of health-related quality of life. Although the cause of their disability is not clear, some investigators suggest that physical and psychosocial disability is caused by mechanisms directly attributable to IEI. Others suggest that the disability results, in part, from treatment recommendations, which can foster illness behavior. Psychological-based factors, i.e., somatic preoccupation, strong illness belief, and resistance to psychological explanations of illness, also could contribute to increased health services utilization and to functional impairment of persons diagnosed with IEI.

SUMMARY

This review demonstrates the robust connection between IEI and psychiatric disorders. Data from both clinical and epidemiologic samples are consistent in showing that persons diagnosed with (or meeting criteria for) IEI frequently suffer from emotional and psychological distress, especially mood, anxiety, somatoform, and personality disorders. They do not appear to be at risk for substance use disorders, psychoses, or antisocial personality disorder.

Proponents of IEI argue that psychiatric problems are a consequence of having a chronic, disabling disorder, and that depression or anxiety is an understandable consequence of IEI. But this argument does not explain the variety of disorders found (each with its own etiologic mechanisms), the increased burden of mental illness in relatives, or the fact that persons diagnosed with IEI are more likely than controls to have preexisting mental illness, a relationship confirmed in clinical studies and in the study of Iowa PGW veterans. In the latter study, though prior psychiatric illness was not specifically assessed, veterans with IEI were more likely than others to have a history of professional psychiatric treatment and prior psychotropic drug usage. The implication of this data is that persons with mental disorders are being misdiagnosed with IEI because their symptoms are misinterpreted as evidence of IEI, or that persons with mental illness are more vulnerable to accepting unproven theories of medical illness.

Finally, the relationship of IEI and psychiatric disorder is important to recognize because it alerts clinicians to the fact that many persons diagnosed with IEI suffer emotional distress and suffer impaired quality of life. Clinicians must fully assess these patients for psychiatric disorders and provide appropriate treatment. Many persons diagnosed with IEI suffer common mental disorders, such as depression or panic disorder, which go untreated, serving to reinforce and exacerbate illness-related disability.

REFERENCES

1. American College of Physicians: Clinical Ecology: Position statement. Ann Intern Med 111:168–178, 1989.
2. American Medical Association: A report of the Council on Scientific Affairs: Clinical Ecology. JAMA 268:3465–3467, 1992.
3. Amundsen MA, Hansen MP, Bruce BK, et al.: Odor aversion or multiple chemical sensitivities; recommendation for a name change and description of successful behavioral medicine treatment. Reg Tox Pharmacol 24:S116–S118, 1996.
4. Barsky AJ, Goodson JD, Lane RS, et al: The amplification of somatic symptoms. Psychosom Med 50:510–519, 1988.
5. Bell IR, Petersen JM, Schwartz GE: Medical histories and psychological profiles of middle-aged women with and without self-reported illness from environmental chemicals. J Clin Psychiatry 56:151–160, 1995.
6. Bell IR, Schwartz GE, Hardin EE, et al.: Differential resting quantitative electroencephalographic alpha patterns in women with environmental intolerance, depressives and normals. Biol Psychiatry 43:376–388, 1998.
7. Binkley KE, Kutcher S: Panic response to sodium lactate infusion in patients with multiple chemical sensitivity syndrome. J Allergy Clin Immunol 99;570–574, 1997.
8. Black DW: Iatrogenic (physician-induced) hypochondriasis—Four patient examples of "chemical sensitivity." Psychosomatics 37:390-393, 1996.
9. Black DW, Sparks PJ: Psychiatric aspects of "chemical sensitivity" syndromes. In Stoudemire A, Vogel B (eds): Medical Psychiatric Practice, Vol. 3. Washington, DC, American Psychiatric Press, pp 347–380, 1995.
10. Black DW, Okiishi C, Gabel J, Schlosser S: Psychiatric illness in the first-degree relatives of persons reporting multiple chemical sensitivities. Tox Indus Health 15:410–414, 1999.
11. Black DW, Rathe A, Goldstein RB: Environmental illness—A controlled study of 26 subjects with "twentieth century disease." JAMA 264:3166–3170, 1990.
12. Black DW, Doebbeling BN, Voelker MD, et al.: Quality of life and health services utilization in a population-based sample of military personnel reporting multiple chemical sensitivities. J Occup Med 41:928–933, 1999.
13. Black DW, Rathe A, Goldstein RB: Measures of distress in 26 "environmentally ill" subjects. Psychosomatics 34;131–138, 1993.
14. Black DW, Doebbeling BN, Voelker, MD, et al.: Multiple chemical sensitivity syndrome: Symptom prevalence and risk factors in a military population. Presented at a meeting sponsored by the Centers for Disease Control and Prevention, Atlanta, GA, February 1999.
15. Black DW, Okiishi C, Schlosser S: A 9-year follow-up of persons diagnosed with multiple chemical sensitivities. Presented at a meeting of the American Chemical Association, Boston, MA, August 1998.
16. Bola-Wilson K, Wilson RJ, Bleeker ML: Conditioning of physical symptoms after neurotoxic exposure. J Occup Med 30:684–686, 1988.
17. Brodsky C: Allergic to everything: A medical subculture. Psychosomatics 24:731–742, 1983.
18. Butcher JN: The Minnesota Report: Adult clinical system MMPI-2. Minneapolis, MN, University of Minnesota Press, 1989.
19. Cullen MR: The worker with multiple chemical sensitivities: An overview. Occup Med 2:655–667, 1997.
20. Davidoff AL, Fogarty L: Psychogenic origins of multiple chemical sensitivities syndrome: A critical review of the research literature. Arch Environ Health 49:316–325, 1994.
21. Derogatis LR: Symptom-Checklist-90-Revised: Administration, Scoring, and Procedures Manual. Towson, MD, Clinical Psychometric Research, 1977.
22. Fiedler N, Maccia C, Kipen H: Evaluation of chemically sensitive patients. J Occup Med 34:529–538, 1992.
23. Fiedler N, Kipen HM, DeLuca J, et al.: A controlled comparison of multiple chemical sensitivities and chronic fatigue syndrome. J Occup Med 52:529–538, 1996.
24. Gothe CJ, Molin C, Nilsson CG: The environmental somatization syndrome. Psychosomatics 36:1–11, 1995.
25. Graveling RA, Pilkington A, George JPK, et al.: A review of multiple chemical sensitivity. Occup Environ Med 56:73–85, 1999.
26. Hyler SE, Reider RO, Spitzer RL: Personality Diagnostic Questionnaire. New York: NY State Psychiatric Institute, 1983.
27. Iowa Persian Gulf Study Group: Self-reported illness and health status among Gulf War veterans. JAMA 277:238–245, 1997.

28. International Program on Chemical Safety: Conclusions and recommendations of a workshop on multiple chemical sensitivities (MCS), Feb. 21-21, Berlin, Germany. Regul Toxicol Pharmacol 24:S188–S189, 1996.
29. Kurt TL: Multiple chemical sensitivities—A syndrome of pseudotoxicity manifested as exposure-perceived symptoms. Clin Toxicol 33:101–105, 1995.
30. Lax MN, Henneberger PK: Patients with multiple chemical sensitivities in an occupational health clinic: Presentation and follow-up. Archives Environ Health 50:425–431, 1995.
31. Leznoff A: Provocative challenges in patients with multiple chemical sensitivity. J Allergy Clin Immunol 99:438–442, 1997.
32. Meggs WJ, Dunn KA, Bloch RM, et al.: Prevalence and nature of allergy and chemical sensitivity in a general population. Arch Environ Health 51:275–282, 1996.
33. Pilowsky I, Spense ND: Manual for the Illness Behavior Questionnaire, 2nd ed. Adelaide, Australia, Dept. of Psychiatry, University of Adelaide, 1983.
34. Robins LN, Helzer JE, Croughan J, Ratcliff KS: The NIMH 'Diagnostic Interview Schedule': Its history, characteristics, and validity. Arch Gen Psychiatry 138:381–389, 1981.
35. Rosenberg SJ, Friedman MR, Schmaling KB, et al.: Personality styles of patients asserting environmental illness. J Occup Med 32:678–681, 1990.
36. Schottenfeld RS: Workers with multiple chemical sensitivities—A psychiatric approach to diagnosis and treatment. Occup Med 2:739–753, 1987.
37. Simon GE, Katon WJ, Sparks PJ: Allergic to life: Psychological factors in environmental illness. Am J Psychiatry 147:901–906, 1990.
38. Simon GE, Daniel LW, Stockbridge H, et al.: Immunologic, psychological and neuropsychological factors in multiple chemical sensitivity—A controlled study. Arch Intern Med 18:97–103, 1993.
39. Shusterman DJ, Dager SR: Prevention of psychological disability after occupational respiratory exposures. Occup Med 6:11–27, 1991.
40. Spitzer RL, Williams JBW, Gibbon M: Structured Clinical Interview for DSM-IV. New York, NY, State Psychiatric Institute, Biometrics Research, 1994.
41. Stangl D, Pfohl B, Zimmerman M, et al: Structured interview for DSM-III personality disorders. Arch Gen Psychiatry 42:591–596, 1985.
42. Staudenmeyer H: Adult sequelae of childhood abuse presenting as environmental illness. Ann Allergy 73:538–546, 1993.
43. Stenn P, Binkley K: Successful outcome in a patient with chemical sensitivity. Psychosomatics 39:547–550, 1998.
44. Stewart DE, Raskin J: Psychiatric assessment of patients with "twentieth century disease" ("total allergy syndrome"). Can Med Asso J 133:1001–1006, 1985.
45. Terr AI: Environmental illness: A clinical review of 50 cases. Arch Intern Med 46:145–149, 1986.
46. Terr AI: Clinical ecology in the workplace. J Occup Med 31:257–261, 1989.
47. Van Valkenberg C, Lowry M, Winokur G, Cadoret R: Depression spectrum disease vs. pure depressive disease. J Nerv Ment Dis 165:341–347, 1977.
48. Ware J: Appendix C. Script for personal interview SF-36 administration. In: SF-36 Health Survey Manuals and Interpretation Guide. Boston, MA, Nimrod Press, 1993.
49. Winokur G: The validity of neurotic-reactive depression. Arch Gen Psychiatry 42:1116–1121, 1985.
50. Witorsch P, Ayesu K, Balter NJ, Schwartz SL: Multiple chemical sensitivity: Clinical features and causal analysis in 61 cases. Presented at the North American Congress on Clinical Toxicology, Rochester, NY, September, 1995.

MICHAEL HODGSON, MD, MPH

SICK BUILDING SYNDROME

From the National Institute of
  Occupational Safety and Health
Washington DC

Reprint requests to:
Michael Hodgson, MD, MPH
NIOSH
Office of the Director
RM 715H, HHH Bldg
200 Independence Avenue SW
Washington DC 20201

The opinions and assertions
contained herein are the views of
the authors and are not to be
construed as the official policy or
position of the United States
government.

The term "sick building syndrome" has been used for 20 years without an operational definition.[33] Nevertheless, attempts to provide alternative names, i.e., problem buildings, building-related occupant complaint syndrome (BROCS), abused building syndrome, and many others, have not met with success, and the term remains in common use. Attempts at defining alternatives reveal two major confusions: (1) Which is the primary concern and problem—the buildings or the occupants? (2) Is the issue the worker's sick feelings and dysfunctional appearance, or are problems objectively measurable?

These confusions distract from the knowledge we do have about human complaints related to the indoor environment and prevent some interested parties from asking the more important questions about mechanisms and prevention. Although empiric data are available for both questions, the data frequently are discussed without an attempt at synthesis. The controversy over the syndrome of idiopathic environmental entolerance (IEI), or multiple chemical sensitivity (MCS), appears to wallow in a similar trap. In fact, the critical questions leading to explicit hypotheses appear quite similar for both syndromes, at least as far as the physiologic effects are concerned. Many practitioners experience patients with the label IEI/MCS as distinct from the vast majority of patients with building-related complaints. Recent data suggest that complaints labeled IEI/MCS are quite common.[43,47] Nevertheless, quantitative approaches based on questionnaire descriptions may fail to capture essential components of the doctor-patient or patient-healthcare provider relationship that defines IEI/MCS.

This chapter summarizes what we know about human symptoms and discomfort in the built environment and formulates several critical hypotheses that show striking parallels to the questions arising from discussions of the syndrome of IEI/MCS. Although the questions are similar, the tone of discussion about MCS often reflects strong beliefs of the discussants, who frequently fail to include major portions of information from the peer-reviewed literature. It is tempting to speculate that the parallels and divergence in opinions about sick building syndrome (SBS) and MCS/IEI reflect physicians' and other scientists' beliefs about and attitudes toward patients and clients, rather than merely the underlying science. In the clinical world this has been called countertransference,[83] and could be explored in a scientific fashion. In addition to published, quantitative data on symptoms considered to comprise SBS, this author has encountered individual patients with symptoms related to low levels of exposure that may fit some criteria for either of two syndromes. These observations (described below) may serve to sharpen the focus of questioning.

THE SPECTRUM OF PATIENTS

Case 1: A 53-year-old design engineer, with both a successful consulting practice and direct responsibility for a major hospital in the mid-West, described confusion and eye irritation whenever he was in laboratories with low levels of exposure to xylene and other solvents. These symptoms had been present for over 20 years. No over-exposures could be identified in his occupational history. He had no chronic diseases. As he was able to control his environment, and rarely entered laboratories, this did not pose a problem to him in his activities of daily living and working.

Case 2: A 55-year old administrative assistant in a courthouse in western Pennsylvania described mucosal irritation, associated with odors of solvents, occurring regularly at work. Air from an engine repair shop in her building circulated into her space through wall perforations. In addition, the ventilation system did not deliver 20 cubic feet of outside air per occupant per minute (cfm) to her space. Over time, her mucosal irritation was accompanied by headaches. Despite intervention by her supervising judge, the building owner was unwilling to bring the space up to professional design specifications. The patient left work. Her symptoms recurred when exposed to strong odors and low levels of solvents and interfered with her ability to work and in her private life.

Case 3: A 35-year-old mother of three children developed generalized mucosal irritation and headaches around the use of a furnace at home. Detailed assessment of the home revealed no cross-contamination or flu entrainment of furnace exhaust gases. She identified a relationship between being at home surrounded by odors and the home where she was sexually abused as a child in a fashion that outlined a therapeutic need. The new sense of danger and "exposedness" in her current home presented therapeutic opportunities. Although she was clearly affected by her illness, after some discussions of leaving the suburban area in which she worked and moving to Montana, she was able to continue in her life activities. Her symptoms did not resolve completely.

Case 4: An executive assistant in a major law firm experienced mucosal irritation and headaches after exposure to paints during painting of occupied space, cleaning with specific agents in her space, and exposure to furniture oils that were used regularly. The global ventilation rate to the building was adequate (approximately 20 cfm oa), and the area of her desk was sparsely occupied. The office management was unwilling to change its strategies of using cleaning agents and renovating because a well-known major indoor environment firm had told them they were "bringing in enough outside air."

These four cases outline critical questions:
- When is occupied space, or the ambient environment, "acceptable" for human occupancy?
- Are there formal criteria levels for specific pollutants below which we do not expect effects?
- Are "low" levels of pollutants defined well enough that we can state when the substances are below levels expected to cause health effects?
- Can common point sources generate exposures that are adequate to lead to adverse health effects?
- How do we define "adverse health effects?"
- Is there objective evidence that individuals with symptoms have physiologic evidence for these symptoms?

Although the psychological contribution to symptoms, and disease in general, is of paramount importance in primary care, a critical examination of the determinants of feeling ill or well; the personality styles and characteristics associated with states of health; the influence of work stress and organizational function (or dysfunction); and the social and legal environment that defines disability in the United States goes beyond the page limitations of this chapter. Work organization, the perception and induction of stress in the work environment, and personality characteristics that lead to specific responses all may be important determinants of the boundary between the two syndromes, if they are different.

SYMPTOMS AND THE BUILT ENVIRONMENT

It is instructive to view the evolution of building complaints from the perspective of occupants empirically and contrast that with the engineering perspective of systems and their evolution.

People

Around the time of the first use of the term SBS, studies strove not merely to describe but also to identify causal relationships. Some clearly identified exposures related to symptoms;[41] others clearly recognized diseases.[8,19] In fact, problems associated with formaldehyde, cleaning agents, moisture, and **bioaerosols** were recognized and well defined. Associations with the complex mixtures that comprise typical indoor pollutant exposures and their potential control through ventilation also were well defined.[73] In fact, one of the early reviews[42] suggested that "traditional industrial hygiene approaches" were unsuccessful. However, thoughtful, innovative, critical investigators generally have been able to identify problems and solve them. Many investigators believe that once specific causes have been identified, the problem under investigation should no longer be called SBS.

Most investigators incorporated "work-relatedness," i.e., that symptoms be "building-related," or improve when away from work, into their case definitions. Nevertheless, it is meanwhile clear that some individuals develop similar problems in the home; 25–50% of complainers describe their symptoms as not being work-related. In addition, in comparisons of two of the commonly used questionnaires,[6] there was only poor agreement on temporal patterns between the two instruments. If some individuals are more susceptible to pollutant effects, then defining only "work-related" symptoms as being of interest and including individuals with persistent symptoms in the control or comparison groups may lead to the introduction of biases in statistical analyses.

Several fundamentally different strategies have been pursued in documenting symptoms. The most widely recognized literature describes symptom prevalence in units of frequency over a time denominator of months or years.[10,20,49,63] These studies generally have failed to identify relationships between symptoms and environmental measures. A separate strategy has been pursued in attempts to document relationships and the effectiveness of interventions,[27,28,82] and these studies have identified relationships between symptoms and a range of exposures, including particulates, low relative humidity, and **volatile organic compounds** (VOC). Finally, some investigators have pursued evidence of physiologic markers of ocular[21,22,37] and nasal physiology.[55,56,79] These document an objective basis for the mucosal irritation that is commonly considered an integral part of the syndrome.

One set of investigations has suggested inter-relationships among the symptom groupings, with mucosal symptoms far more strongly related to each other than to other symptoms.[27] Several basic mechanisms may then be involved in the generation of complaints among office workers, in part across organs. The common chemical sense, based on predictable dose-response relationships of the irritant receptor, may be involved in eye and nose irritation.[12] Some evidence supports traditional allergy as contributing to at least some portion of nasal symptoms.[45,50] In fact, even headaches appear to be more frequent in allergy sufferers in office environments.[45] It is clear that objective measures of personal susceptibility are related both to increased symptom rates[65] and to symptoms at lower exposure levels.[38]

Two separate research directions evolved, one generally supporting the bioaerosols hypothesis, the other the VOC hypothesis. These two hypotheses postulate specific triggers for discomfort and health symptoms that work stress and thermal discomfort may exaggerate.

BIOAEROSOLS

In the course of searching for moisture and humidifier fever[5] in buildings, Finnegan et al. Found that symptoms were associated with **humidification and ventilation**.[20] Subsequently other early, large-scale investigations identified a high prevalence of symptoms belonging to a range of organs and potential mechanisms.[10,63]

Cross-sectional studies subsequently have supported an association of higher rates of symptoms with endotoxin exposure[70] and with the presence of unwanted moisture in ventilation systems.[61] A small portion of individuals with building-related nasal complaints appear to have allergies to specific agents identified in their building.[50] In addition, individuals with IgE antibodies to agents commonly found in buildings appear to have more symptoms than do individuals without such antibodies.[45] On the other hand, Kjaergard[38] showed that individuals with atopy reacted to a defined concentration of a complex VOC mixture at substantially lower concentrations than controls without atopy. Similarly, Shusterman[58a] demonstrated that atopic individuals decrease their nasal airway resistance substantially more than nonatopic individuals after a challenge with chlorine.

Several recent case reports have identified building moisture as associated with symptoms that are poorly understood but may represent some immunological effect.[30,35] In fact, in one recent study, a building with a single confirmed case of hypersensitivity pneumonitis had a substantially elevated rate of "nonspecific" symptoms (which also were consistent with hypersensitivity pneumonitis), but failed to show any objective evidence of disease in patients.[77] These reports suggest that symptom excess in the presence of moisture represents some phenomenon related to bioaerosols exposure.

VOLATILE ORGANIC COMPOUNDS

Investigators in Denmark[22,23,39,52] pursued the hypothesis that complex mixtures of volatile organic compounds might be the primary cause of mucosal irritation, a prominent symptom, and that these agents might also contribute to headaches, fatigue, and dizziness. The associated, though generally unspoken, accompanying hypothesis was that these agents were recognized as a cause of solvent neurotoxicity at higher concentrations and that dose-response relationships with less severe forms of disease were simply not well understood.[52]

Evidence exists that volatile organic compounds are important in occupant complaints in large buildings. Chamber studies have demonstrated associations,[31,52] although more recent, smaller studies have not replicated the results. Several field studies demonstrated associations. Hodgson et al.[27] demonstrated a univariate relationship between VOCs measured with a flame ionization detector. Hodgson et al.,[28] using a VOC measurement method with substantially greater imprecision, showed relationships between VOCs and mucosal irritation after controlling for perceptions of work stress. Sundell demonstrated an association of symptoms with decreases in VOC concentrations from supply to exhaust air within rooms,[66,67] suggesting that the mechanism identified by Wechsler termed "indoor chemistry" leads to "lost VOCs" and is associated with mucosal irritation. The topic recently has been reviewed.[3] Brinke suggested an association between symptom groupings and VOCs clustered by likely source.[69]

Cain and Cometto-Muniz[12] have conducted a series of chamber studies documenting predictable dose-response relationships between homologous series of alcohols, acids, and aldehydes and stimulating the common chemical sense, i.e., the irritant receptor. Abraham et al.[1] used these to develop a quantitative structure activity relatiionship that allows the prediction of irritation based on the physical characteristics of the molecules. At least at concentrations in the vicinity of the irritant threshold, the dose-response relationships support simple dose-additivity.[15a] The nature of such relationships at concentrations well below irritant thresholds remains to be clarified fully. Alarie et al.[2] demonstrated that some "reactive" species trigger symptoms that do not follow this predictable pattern, and that, therefore, reactive species must act through a different mechanism. In addition to simple triggering of a receptor, irritation also may .arise from chemical reactions in the mucosa.

Wechsler[75,76] suggested one mechanism by which more potent irritation may be induced in indoor environments than would be expected from the usual agents encountered indoors. The presence of reactive species, of ozone for example, allows the formation of **Criegee radicals** and **the oxidation of less reactive species to aldehydes**. In the presence of air exchange rates of more than 1 air exchange per hour and ozone levels above 0.1 ppm, aldehyde levels are likely to be irritating to office occupants.

In one investigation of hospitals, moisture-associated deterioration of building materials was found to lead to elevated exposures of irritants,[78] although this is disputed by some because concentrations of relatively inert VOCs do not reach irritant concentrations.

Critical to this discussion is the fact that a dose-related increase in symptoms does appear at levels one to two orders of magnitude below permissible exposure levels and threshold limit values. These relationships support population-based studies suggesting that the presence of widespread symptoms is not implausible simply because "exposures are below all permissible levels." In recognition of this observation, concentration levels recommended for indoor environments generally are substantially lower than those relied upon in the occupational hygiene field (Table 1).

TABLE 1.   Comparison of Guidelines and Standards Pertinent to Indoor Environments[a]

	Canadian	WHO/Europe	NAAQS/EPA	SMAC	NIOSH REL	OSHA	ACGIH	MAK
Formaldehyde	0.1 ppm [L] 0.05 ppm [L][b]	0.081 ppm [30 m]			0.016 ppm 0.1 ppm [15m]	0.75 ppm 2 ppm [15m]	0.3 ppm [C]	0.5 ppm 1 ppm [5m]
Carbon dioxide	3,500 ppm [L]				5,000 ppm 30,000 ppm [15m]	10,000 ppm 30,000 ppm [15m]	5,000 ppm 30,000 ppm [15m]	5,000 ppm 10,000 ppm [1h]
Carbon monoxide[c]	11 ppm [8h] 25 ppm [1h]	87 ppm [15m] 52 ppm [30m] 26 ppm [1h] 8.7 ppm [8h]	9 ppm[g] 35 ppm [1h][g]		35 ppm 200 ppm [C]	35 ppm 200 ppm [5m] 1500 [C]	25 ppm	30 ppm 60 ppm [30m]
Nitrogen dioxide	0.05 ppm 0.25 ppm [1h]	0.2 ppm [1h] 0.08 ppm [24h]	0.05 ppm [1y]		1 ppm [15m]	1 ppm [15m]	3 ppm 5 ppm [15m]	5 ppm 10 ppm [5m]
Ozone	0.12 ppm [1h]	0.08–0.1 ppm [1h] 0.05–0.06 ppm [8h]	0.12 ppm [1h] 0.08 ppm [8h]		0.1 ppm [C]	0.1 ppm 0.3 ppm [15m]	0.05 ppm 0.2 ppm [15m]	0.1 ppm 0.2 ppm [5m]
Particles[e] < 2.5 MMAD[d]	0.1 mg/m³ [1h] 0.040 mg/m³ [L]					5 mg/m³	3 mg/m³	
Particles[e] < 10 MMAD[d]			0.05 mg/m³ [1y] 0.15 mg/m³ [24h][g]				10 mg/m³	
Total particles[e]						15 µg/m³		
Sulfur dioxide	0.38 ppm [5m] 0.019 ppm	0.19 ppm [10m] 0.13 ppm [1h]	0.03 ppm [1y] 0.14 ppm [24h][g]		2 ppm 5 ppm [15m]	2 ppm 5 ppm [15m]	2 ppm 5 ppm [15m]	2 ppm 4 ppm [5m]
Lead	Minimize exposure	0.5–1.0 µg/m³ [1y]	1.5 µg/m³ 3 months		< 0.1 mg/m³ [10h]	0.05 mg/m³	0.05 mg/m³	0.1 mg/m³ 1 mg/m³ [30m]
Radon	2.7 pCi/L [1y]		4 pCi/L [L][f]					2 ppm 4 ppm [5m]

This table was prepared with Hal Levin for an appendix of Standard 62 ("Ventilation for Acceptable Air Quality") and Guideline Project Committee 10 within the standards development process at the American Society for Heating, Refrigerating, and Airconditioning Engineers.

(Table notes continued on next page.)

[ ] Numbers in brackets refer to either a ceiling or to averaging times of less than or greater to 8 hours (m = minutes; h = hours; y = year; C = ceiling, L = long-term) Where no time is specified, the averaging time is 8 hours.

a **The values summarized in this table include:**
- Canadian: Recommended maximum exposures for residences developed in 1987 by a committee of Provincial members convened by the federal government to establish consensus, "guideline"-type levels. A revised version is being considered. These were not designed to be enforceable. They were designed explicitly for the residential environment.
- WHO/Europe: Environmental (non-industrial) guidelines developed in 1987 by the WHO Office for Europe (Denmark).
- NAAQS: Criteria for outdoor air developed under the Clean Air Act by the US EPA. The guidelines must, by law, be reviewed every five years, although this does not always occur. These levels are ostensibly selected to protect most sensitive individuals. Exposure level may vary by duration of exposure. Sensory irritation was not a consideration in establishing levels.
- NIOSH: Recommended maximum exposures for industrial environments developed by NIOSH (Centers for Disease Control). NIOSH criteria documents contain both a review of the literature and a recommended exposure guideline. Sensory irritation was not a consideration in establishing levels. These are not enforceable and not reviewed regularly. These levels are not selected to protect most sensitive individuals.
- OSHA: Enforceable maximum exposures for industrial environments developed by OSHA (US Department of Labor) through a standard setting process. Once a standard has been set, levels can be changed only through reopening the rule-making process. These levels are not selected to protect most sensitive individuals. Sensory irritation was not a consideration in establishing levels.
- ACGIH: Recommended maximum exposures for industrial environments developed by ACGIH's Threshold Limit Values Committee. The committee reviews the scientific literature and recommends exposure guidelines. The assumptions are for usual working conditions, 40 hour weeks, and single exposures. These levels are not selected to protect most sensitive individuals. Sensory irritation was not a primary consideration in establishing levels.
- MAK: Recommended maximum exposures for industrial environments developed by the Deutsche Forschungs Gemeinschaft, a German institutions akin to the National Academy of Sciences and Institutes of Health, without regulatory powers. Levels are set on a regular basis, with annual reviews and periodic republication of criteria levels. These levels are enforceable in Germany. These levels are not selected to protect most sensitive individuals. Sensory irritation was not a consideration in establishing levels.
- SMAC: Spacecraft Maximal Allowable Concentrations were developed by a Committee of Toxicology convened by the National Academy of Sciences. They were developed for prolonged exposure periods with consideration of continuous (24 hours per day) exposure. The Committee Report was funded by NASA.

b Target level of .05 ppm because of its carcinogenic effects. Total aldehydes limited to 1 ppm.

c As one example, readers should consider the applicability of carbon monoxide concentrations. The concentrations considered acceptable for non-industrial, as opposed to industrial occupational, exposure are substantially lower. This is due to the recognition that individuals with pre-existing heart disease may develop exacerbation of heart disease at levels below 15 ppm.

d MMAD = mass median aerodynamic diameter in microns (micrometers). Less than 2.5 mm are considered respirable; less than 10 mm are considered inhalable.

e Nuisance particles not otherwise classified, not known to contain significant amounts of asbestos, lead, crystalline silica, known carcinogens, or other particles known to cause significant adverse health effects.

f The U.S. EPA has promulgated a guideline value of 4 pCi/L indoor concentration. This is not a regulatory value but an action level where mitigation is recommended if the value is exceeded in long-term tests.

g Not to be exceeded more than once per year.

The four major questions to be considered in relying on the data from this table are:

- Does the standard aim to prevent the effect of concern in the setting in which it is being used?
- Does the standard recognize the presence of susceptible groups or address the "normal" population?
- Are interactions between various contaminants of concern considered?
- Are the assumptions and conditions set forth by the standard met (such as 8-hour day, 40-hour work week)?

At times, the selection of a specific target level is best made by a team with wide experience in toxicology, industrial hygiene, and exposure assessment.

INDIVIDUAL SUSCEPTIBILITY

Investigations on the physiology of mucosal irritation in buildings suggested that individuals with building-related complaints had, as a group, more rapid tear film break-up time and were more likely to suffer from punctate conjunctivitis.[22,23] It is unclear whether these effects represent a marker of susceptibility, a consequence of exposure, or a mechanism. Tsubota[71] has reviewed the physiology of tear film production and suggests two mechanisms by which underlying susceptibility might increase eye complaints. First, both decreased basal and reflex stimulation lead to dry eye complaints. In addition, decreased Meibomian gland lipid secretion will allow more rapid evaporation of tear fluid in the presence of enlarged exposed ocular surface during computer screen work.[72]

Although some work suggests that individuals with building-related nasal complaints have increased nasal reactivity,[55,56] as a group such subjects do not demonstrate decrements in nasal volume[6] (Roberts, personal communication).

Kjaergard and coauthors have presented evidence from chamber studies that atopic individuals may be more susceptible to the irritant effects of VOCs at low concentrations. They documented that atopic individuals describe more severe irritation at lower thresholds than do nonatopics.[38,39]

Stenberg suggested that subjects with dermal complaints were more likely to describe eczema and to describe more severe irritation on a standardized test of dermal response to a dilute acid ("stinger test") than individuals without complaints.[65]

HEADACHES, STRESS, AND THERMAL DISCOMFORT

Headaches are recognized as a common symptom among office workers,[59,60] though these generally have not been classified into standard categories.[32] In addition, many employers have moved beyond the passive counting of complaints into interventions and have demonstrated several successful intervention programs directed at individuals.[58] It remains unclear how headache proneness, work-relatedness, and the social and organizational aspects of work contribute to the development of complaints.

Since the early part of this century, engineers have recognized that thermal discomfort is a major contributor to indoor environmental complaints. Flugge demonstrated that odor perception and heat sensation were the main reasons for ventilating occupied space.[34] Subsequent empiric work has confirmed that the thermal comfort envelope does not provide an adequate margin of "comfort" when other modalities of exposure approach their own acceptability boundaries.

Finally, it is hard to consider occupant discomfort and symptoms in the built environment without acknowledging that all discomfort and disease have a psycholgic component. It is clear that symptoms are strongly associated with psy-chological factors.[18,49] As importantly, work stress appears to explain a greater pro-portion of the variance of symptoms than do the measured exposures.[28] This may simply reflect our much more robust ability to characterize work stress and our lack of knowledge about specific exposure assessment techniques, than a true stronger relationship.

Engineering Aspects of Buildings

Engineers have been concerned about the requirements for ventilation in occu-pied space since the last 19th century. Although some considerations occurred ear-lier, as von Pettenkofer used carbon dioxide as a marker of ventilation requirements, the first formal, scientifically derived standard was suggested in 1892 by Billings.

Jansen[34] recently reviewed the history of ventilation. The first issue of the Transaction of the American Society for Ventilating Engineers in the 1890s sug-gested the need for 30 cubic feet of outside air per occupant per minute, primarily to prevent disease transmission . Odors and heat were recognized as distinct discom-fort-inducing environmental parameters by Flugge in the early part of this century. Subsequently, chamber experiments in Yaglou's laboratory in Boston in the 1920s and 1930s documented the need for ventilation for odor control and the increased ventilation requirements for environmental tobacco smoke comfort.

The American Society for Heating, Refrigerating, and Air-Conditioning Engineers (ASHRAE) promulgated its ventilation standard in 1972. Subsequently the "energy crisis" led to a reduction in recommended ventilation rates. Recognizing that these 5 cfm oa were simply inadequate where tobacco smoking was permitted, venti-lation requirements were raised in the presence of smoking. The ensuing controversy, and pressure from various parties, led to a delay in the next revision until 1989, when version 62-89 maintained that all buildings should be ventilated at 20 cfm oa per oc-cupant, and, hidden in a footnote, that "this addresses a small amount of smoking." When continuing controversy prevented the issuance of an updated version, the stan-dard went into "continuous maintenance." As new knowledge emerges, it is incorpo-rated without rewriting the whole standard. The smoking footnote has been removed. There is agreement that buildings need at 20 cfm oa to remove usual human odors and emissions and that strong sources require more ventilation.

Thermal comfort standards have been developed in a series of chamber stud-ies beginning with the Pierce Foundation studies in the 1920s. There is clear over-lap between the expression of thermal discomfort and mucosal irritation, as with other domains of symptoms. Temperatures in buildings with complaints often exceed the recommended thermal envelope. In addition, the thermal comfort en-velopes for women and men do not completely coincide, so that individuals of one gender may express, on average, discomfort when individuals of the other gender feel satisfied.

Although engineering models are developed and refined on the basis of empiri-cal evidence, the theoretical derivations generally are incorporated into voluntary professional design standards, which are then used on a daily basis. Although the science of engineering represents a complex interplay between empirically derived standards and sophisticated theoretical thinking, the daily practice of engineering is far more mundane. Even though buildings may have, on balance, adequate ventila-tion, air often is distributed in nonuniform fashion to the spaces within buildings, leading to local outdoor air deficits. Similarly, retrofits, additional thermal loads from machines (computers), and office redesign may lead to local thermal loads in excess of design. Similarly, although most trades have standardized approaches to doing things (captured in apprenticeship courses, codes, and manuals), a recent conference (Bugs, Mold, and Rot III 1999) recognized that the daily practice of construction may lag far behind the state of knowledge inherent in standards.

Data on the problems in buildings have been recognized over the years, beginning with early NIOSH attempts to classify the single most important factor causing problems.[48] The first International Conference on Indoor Air Quality and Climate, now a triennial conference series, was held in 1978. In recognition, ASHRAE instituted an Environmental Health Committee and an annual indoor air quality meeting. Several investigators documented that most buildings suffered from more than one deficiency, with the single most common problem being ventilation systems.[80] This included inadequate provision of outside air, inadequate distribution to occupied space, and inadequate filtration. Almost more importantly, the majority of building maintenance personnel in buildings with problems did not understand how the systems under their control had been designed and were to be operated. Ten years later at least outside air delivery may have improved,[15] though the techniques in such studies differ so dramatically that this may represent a wishful interpretation.

ARE THE SYNDROMES DIFFERENT?

Jaakola[33] has argued that the lack of an operational definition reflects the widespread recognition that the "syndrome" represents a theoretical construct for discussion purposes only. As outlined above, a broad range of symptoms has been attributed to the indoor environment, and a series of physiologic measures suggest several different mechanisms involved in the etiology of those symptoms. Exposures to bioaerosols and VOCs have been associated with symptoms. It is not likely that all symptom categories are caused by a single mechanism, or that a single pollutant class causes all problems. A major issue remains in discussions of SBS: that no operational definition exists and that there is not even agreement on whether individuals can suffer from "the" problem or whether it represents a simple quantitative problem definable only in groups.

Lack of Operational Definitions

Does the presence of regular eye irritation, with or without punctate conjunctivitis, in a single occupant represent SBS if there are a total of five regular building occupants? Four? Six? Some professionals have argued for a 20% cut-off threshold. If we acknowledge that there is a quantitative frequency threshold, for example of 20% prevalence, how often must such symptoms occur for them to count toward the syndrome? Every day? Most days of the week? Three or more days per week? Most weeks? On average one day per week? In any case, most scientists agree that buildings must be occupied and some proportion of individuals must complain for the label to have relevance.

SBS may be dealt with on three levels: **office workers who are sick, the building systems, and the work process itself**. This approach reflects a fundamental belief in occupational health, in which work, the worker, and the workplace are considered as three distinct, but key, ingredients.[65] The latter represents not just the work process in the physical sense—with engineering generation and control strategies—but also the social and organizational structure in the workplace. Unless problems are addressed at all three levels, it is hard to come to understand the processes or to intervene effectively. In a topic such as this, the true etiology is of interest because it may lead to intervention strategies in specific buildings as well as on an individual level, and, in the long run, it may guide engineering strategies.

This model also implies that organizational intervention is necessary and appropriate. The formation of air quality teams or committees in many buildings, the structure of the proposed indoor air standard from the Occupational Safety and Health Administration, and experience suggest the importance.

These strategies contrast dramatically with those of IEI/MCS: individuals develop a problem; the individual is labeled as being ill. Some might argue the distinction reflects professionals' beliefs and knowledge, rather than any specific scientific understanding, and guides intervention strategies.

What Do We Mean by Low Levels?

Many practitioners acknowledge that indoor environments generate pollutant concentrations "well below OSHA standards" and that these concentrations are nevertheless associated with effects. Less well known is how well documented "low-level" effects are or how widely held such views are even in the scientific community. The most complex issue remains that of VOCs. Much of the scientific and epidemiologic work on VOCs has been based on mass concentration approaches.[52,74,80] Although the experimental work has suggested dose-response relationships, the work has not led to the development of standards for two reasons. First, the degree of agonism between various agents at levels below their own irritant threshold remains unclear. If low levels of pollutants interact more strongly as there are more agents present, and as they are more lipophilic, many more agents must be studied before a reasonably predictive model of irritation can be established for simple irritation. Second, the presence of reactive species such as ozone can generate agents that cause irritation not just through the common chemical sense but also through other forms of irritation, i.e., direct toxic reactions. This reaction is dependent not just on the mixture of VOCs and the concentrations of the various reactive species, but also on the air exchange rate, which affects the duration that concentrations of reactive species are available for the formation of Criegee radicals and the oxidation to aldehydes. The differences between atopic and nonatopic individuals has been inadequately studied.

Do Low Levels of Exposure Cause Real Health Effects?

Scientists have argued for years about the definition of "health effects" in the indoor environment.[13] Some have argued that "sensations" such as irritation represent purely subjective effects and therefore should not be considered evidence of pathophysiology. On the other hand, irritation is clearly recognized as an effect supported by animal models, large-scale epidemiology, and mechanistic thinking. The 1988 PELs decision, which remanded the Permissible Exposure Levels Project to the Occupational Safety and Health Administration, clearly acknowledged that irritation by itself was a reasonable basis for OSHA standards. Irritation is associated with impaired visual acuity,[57] which is likely a harbinger of decreased productivity and certainly an adverse economic, if not health, effect.

Patients whose symptoms are initially induced by acute irritant exposures may progress to longer term symptoms. The physiologic basis remains unclear. Nevertheless, the various syndromes of "unexplained symptoms" associated with perceived exposure affect larger groups of populations than expected.[43,47,53] At least war-related trauma is associated with earlier death from all causes, not just suicide and motor vehicle accidents,[17,26] and suggests that psychological determinants of well being and long-term mortality health may need to be considered.

Do Markers Exist?

Clinical studies have identified markers of group differences in eye and nasal function after VOC exposure and in association with symptoms. Still, none of these techniques have receiver-operating test characteristic curves that are well developed enough to permit clinical use in diagnosis, with the exception of tear film break-up time and conjunctival staining for punctate conjunctivitis, which is in use in clinical settings and widely available.

It remains unclear how useful tear film break-up time, fluorescent dye staining for punctate conjunctivitis, and other tests will be in distinguishing healthy from affected building occupants and individuals with building-related symptoms from patients with SBS/IEI, or in identifying individuals with an objective basis for IEI/MCS.

SUMMARY

There is reasonable evidence that an objective basis exists for SBS, based on both laboratory and field studies. Intervention strategies for environmental control in the office appear to solve many of the problems, although engineering design strategies sometimes are inadequate. Is there evidence that these data pertain to MCS?

A major problem arises from the missing agreed-upon case definitions for the two conditions. They are similar in that both appear to be due to low levels of agents, well below PELs, TLVs, and other levels established by scientific groups. This similarity may be due to one of two separate mechanisms. First, criteria levels do not appear to protect everyone against effects such as irritation, based on empiric field and laboratory data. Second, data do indicate that some individuals respond to concentrations of agents at levels below such "criteria" levels, because of definable and measurable problems such as atopy or more rapid tear film break-up time. Both syndromes appear to affect different organ systems, or at least be associated with symptoms attributed to different organ systems (mucosal irritation, chest symptoms, nausea, headaches). The problem of resolution after leaving work, or the inciting building, is somewhat more difficult, as questionnaire-based responses do not appear to show strong concordance between the two main questionnaires, administered simultaneously, that are used to define SBS symptoms. Psychological aspects clearly influence interpretations of symptoms in SBS. Although this is documented for some proportion of MCS/IEI, it remains controversial. Psychological aspects of discomfort, and stress, are clearly acknowledged to be important in office worker symptoms, at least as pertains to their magnitude.

Some years ago, the AMA Council of Scientific Affairs used one publication by this author[27] to distinguish the two conditions.[14] In the absence of more formal study, and better case definitions, the scientific evidence summarized here simply provides evidence supporting a physiologic basis for symptoms at very low levels, the influence of psychological states on symptoms, and the presence of reversible dose-related symptoms at levels below defined criteria levels. Still, this author feels uncomfortable equating the two syndromes, experiences patients who have been labeled MCS/IEI differently, and remains unconvinced that the syndromes are indistinguishable.

REFERENCES

  1. Abraham M: Potency of gases and vapors: QSARs. Gammage RB (ed): Indoor Air and Human Health. CITY, Lewis Publishing, 1996.
  2. Alarie Y, Schaper M, Nielsen GD, Abraham MH: Structure-activity relationships of volatile organic chemicals as sensory irritants. Arch Toxicol 1998;72(3):125–140.

3. Anderson K, Bakke J, Bjorseth O, et al: TVOC and health in nonindustrial indoor environments. Report from a Nordic Scientific Consensus Meeting in Stockholm 1996. Indoor Air 1997;7: 78–91.

4. Andersen I, Lundqvist GR, Jensen PL, Proctor DF: Human response to 78-hour exposure to dry air. Arch Environ Health 1974;29:319–324.

5. Anonymous: Humidifier fever revisited. Lancet 1980;1:1286–1287.

6. Apter A, Hodgson M, Lueng W-Y, Pichnarcik L: Nasal symptoms in the "Sick Building Syndrome." (Abstract). Ann Allergy Asthma Immunol 1997;78:152.

7. Barsky AJ, Borus JF: Functional somatic syndromes. Ann Intern Med 1999;130:910–921.

8. Bernstein RS, Sorenson WG, Garabrant D, et al: Exposures to respirable, airborne Penicillium from a contaminated ventilation system: Clinical, environmental, and epidemiological aspects. Am Ind Hyg Assoc J 1983;44:161–169.

9. Boswell T, DiBerardinis, Ducatman A: Descriptive epidemiology of indoor odor complaints at a large teaching institution. Appl Occup Environ Hyg 1994;9:281–286.

10. Burge PS, Hedge A, Wilson S, et al: Sick-building syndrome: A study of 4373 office workers. Ann Occup Hyg 1987;31:493–504.

11. Burge PS, Robertson AS, Hedge A: Comparison of a self-administered questionnaire with physician diagnosis in the diagnosis of the sick building syndrome. Indoor Air 1991;1:422–427.

12. Cain WS: Odors and irritation in indoor air pollution. Gammage RB (ed): Indoor Air and Human Health. CITY, Lewis Publishing, 1996.

13. Cain WS, Samet JM, Hodgson M: The quest for negligible health risk from indoor air. ASHRAE J VOL/ISSUE:PAGES, 1995.

13a. Cain WS, Cometto-Muniz WS, Abraham M, Gola JM: Chemosensory detection of 1-butanol and 2-heptanone in single and binary mixtures. Physiol Behav 1999;67:269–276.

14. Council on Scientific Affairs, American Medical Association: Clinical ecology. JAMA 1992; 268:3465–3467.

15. Crandall M, Sieber W: The National Institute for Occupational Safety and Health Indoor Environmental Evaluation Experience. Part one: Building environmental evaluations. Appl Occup Environ Hyg 1996;11:533–539.

16. deShazo RD, Chapin K, Swain RE: Fungal sinusitis. N Engl J Med 1997;337:254–259.

17. Elder GH, Shanahan MJ, Clipp EC: Linking combat and physical health: The legacy of World War II in men's lives. Am J Psychiatry 1997;154:330–336.

18. Eriksson N, Hoog J, Mild KH, et al: The psychosocial work environment and skin symptoms among visual display terminal workers: A case referent study. Int J Epidemiol 1997;26:1250–1257.

19. Fink JN, Thiede WH, Banaszak EF, Barboriak JJ: Interstitial pneumonitis due to hypersensitivity to an organism contaminating a heating system. Ann Intern Med 1971;74:80–83.

20. Finnegan M, Pickering CAC, Burge PS: The sick-building syndrome: Prevalence studies. Br Med J 1984;289:1573–1575.

21. Fisk W, Rosenfeld AH: Estimates of improved productivity and health from better indoor environments. Indoor Air 1997;7:158–172.

22. Franck C, Bach E, Skov P: Prevalence of objective eye manifestations in people working in office buildings with different prevalences of the sick building syndrome compared with the general population. Int Arch Occup Environ Health 1993;65:65–69.

23. Franck C, Skov P: Foam at inner eye canthus in office workers, compared with an average Danish population as control group. Acta Ophthalmol (Copenh) 1989;67:61–68.

24. Gerrity T, Feussner M: Emerging research on the treatment of Gulf War veterans' illnesses. J Occup Envir Med 1999;41:440–442.

25. Gun RT, Jezukaitis PT: RSI: A perspective from its birthplace. Occup Med 1999;14:81–95.

26. Hearst N, Hulley SB, Newman TB: Delayed effects of the military draft on mortality. A randomized natural experiment. N Engl J Med 1986;314:620–624.

27. Hodgson MJ, Frohliger J, Permar E, et al: Symptoms and microenvironmental measures in non-problem buildings. J Occup Med 1991;33:527–533.

28. Hodgson MJ, Muldoon S, Collopy P, Olesen B: Work stress, symptoms, and microenvironmental measures. Indoor Air Quality 92: Environments for people. ASHRAE, Atlanta, 1992, pp 47–58.

29. Hodgson MJ: A series of field studies on the sick-building syndrome. Ann N Y Acad Sciences 1992;641:21–36.

30. Hodgson MJ, Morey P, Leung W-Y, et al: Pulmonary disease and mycotoxin exposure in Florida associated with *Aspergillus versicolor* and *Stachybotrys atra* exposure. J Occup Environ Med 1998;40:241–249.

31. Hudnell HK, Otto DA, House DE, Molhave L: Exposure of humans to a volatile organic mixture. II. Sensory. Arch Environ Health 1992;47:31–38.

32. International Society for the Study of Headache. Classification Criteria. 1993.
33. Jaakola JJ: The office enviroinment model: A conceptual analysis of the sick building syndrome. Indoor Air 1998 (Suppl 4):7–16.
34. Jansen J: The "V" in AHSVE: A historical perspective. ASHRAE J 1994; 126–132.
35. Johanning E, Biagini R, Hull D, et al: Health and immunology study following exposure to toxigenic fungi (*Stachybotrys chartarum*) in a water-damaged office environment. Int Arch Occup Environ Health 1996;68:207–218.
36. Jones JW, Barge BN, Steffy BD, et al: Stress and medical malpractice: Organizational risk assessment and intervention. J Appl Psychol 1988;73:727–735.
37. Kjaergard S: Assessment methods and causes of eye irritation in humans in indoor environments. Knoeppel H, Wolkoff P (eds): Chemical, microbiological, health, and comfort aspectsof indoor air quality. ECSC, EEC, EAEC, Brussels, 1992;115–127.
38. Kjaergard S, Rasmussen TR, Molhave L, Pedersen OF. An experimental comparison of indoor air VOC effects on hayfever and healthy subjects. Proceedings of Healthy Buildings 95. 1995;1: 564–569.
39. Kjaergaard S, Pedersen OF, Molhave L: Sensitivity of the eyes to airborne irritant stimuli: Influence of individual characteristics. Arch Environ Health 1992;47:45–50.
40. Koren HS, Devlin RB: Human upper respiratory tract responses to inhaled pollutants with emphasis on nasal lavage. Ann N Y Acad Sci 1992;641:215–224.
41. Kreiss K, Gonzalez MG, Conright KL, Schere AR: Respiratory irritation from carpet shampoo. Environment Interna 1982;8:337–342.
42. Kreiss K, Hodgson MJ: Building-associated epidemics. In CS Walsh, Dudney PJ, Copenhaever E (eds): Indoor Air Quality. Boca Raton , CRC Press,1984, pp 87–106.
43. Kreutzer R, Neutra RR, Lashuay N : Prevalence of people reporting sensitivities to chemicals in a population-based survey. Am J Epidemiol 1999;150:1–12.
44. Malkin R, Wilcox T, Sieber W: The National Institute for Occupational Safety and Health Indoor Environmental Evaluation Experience. Part two: Symptom prevalence. Appl Occupl Environ Hygiene 1996;11:540–545.
45. Malkin R, Martinez K, Marinkovich V, et al: The relationship between symptoms and IgG and IgE antibodies in an office environment. Environ Res 1998;76:85–93.
46. Meggs WJ, Albernaz M, Elsheik T, et al: Nasal pathology and ultrastructure in patients with chronic airway inflammation (RADS and RUDS) following an irritant exposure J Toxicol Clin Toxicol 1996;34:383–396.
47. Meggs WJ, Dunn KA, Bloch RM, et al: Prevalence and nature of allergy and chemical sensitivity in a general population. Arch Environ Health 1996;51:275–282.
48. Melius J, Wallingford K, Keenlyside R, Carpenter J: Indoor air quality: The NIOSH experience. Ann Am Conf Gov Indust Hyg 1984;10:3–7.
49. Mendell M: Nonspecific symptoms in office workers: A review and summary of the epidemiologic literature. Indoor Air 1993;3:227–236.
50. Menzies D, Comtois P, Pasztor J, et al: Aeroallergens and work-related respiratory symptoms among office workers. J Allergy Clin Immunol 1998;101:38–44.
51. Molhave L, Liu Z, Jorgensen AH, et al: Sensory and physiologic effects on humans of combined exposures to air temperatures and volatile organic compounds. Indoor Air 1993;3:155–169.
52. Molhave L: Controlled experiments for studies of the sick building syndrome. Ann N Y Acad Sci 1992;641:46–55.
53. Nelson C, Wallace LA, Clayton CA, et al: Indoor air quality and work environment survey: Relationships of employee's self-reported symptoms and direct indoor air quality measurements. Atlanta, Georgia, IAQ 91, ASHRAE, 1991, pp 22–32.
54. Nordstrom K, Norback D, Akselsson R : Effect of air humidification on the sick building syndrome and perceived indoor air quality in hospitals: a four month longitudinal study. Occup Environ Med 1994;51:683–688.
55. Ohm M, Juto JE, Andersson K, Bodin L: Nasal histamine provocation of tenants in a sick-building residential area. Am J Rhinol 1997;11:167–175.
56. Ohm M,Juto JE, Andersson K: Nasal hyperreactivity and sick building syndrome. Atlanta, Georgia, IAQ 92: Environments for People, ASHRAE,1993.
57. Rolando M, Lester M, Macri A, Calabria G: Low spatial-contrast sensitivity in dry eyes. Cornea 1998;17:376–379.
58. Schneider WJ, Furth PA, Blalock TH, Sherrill TA: A pilot study of a headache program in the workplace. The effect of education. J Occup Environ Med 1999;41:202–209.
58a. Shusterman DJ, Murphy MA, Balmes JR: Subjects with seasonal allergic rhinitis react differently to nasal provocation with chlorine gas. J Allergy Clin Immunol 1998;101:732–740.

59. Schwartz BS, Stewart WF, Lipton RB: Lost workdays and decreased work effectiveness associated with headache in the workplace. J Occup Environ Med 1997;39:320–327.

60. Schwartz BS, Stewart WF, Simon D, Lipton RB: Epidemiology of tension-type headache. JAMA 1998;279:381–383.

61. Sieber WK, Stayner LT, Malkin R, et al: The NIOSH indoor evaluation experience: Associations between environmental factors and self-reported health conditions. Appl Occup Environ Hygiene 1996;11:1387–392.

62. See reference 61.

63. Skov P, Valbjorn O, Pedersen BV: Influence of indoor climate on the sick building syndrome in an office environment. The Danish Indoor Climate Study Group. Scand J Work Environ Health 1990;16:363–371.

64. Stenberg B, Wall S: Why do women report 'sick building symptoms' more often than men? Soc Sci Med 1995;40:491–502.

65. Stenberg B: Office illness: The worker, the work, and the workplace. Sweden, NIOH, 1994.

66. Sundell J, Andersson B, Andersson K, Lindvall T: Volatile organic compounds in ventilating air in buildings at different sampling points in the buildings and their relationship with the prevalence of occupant symptoms. Indoor Air 1993;3:82–93.

67. Sundell J: On the association between building ventilation characteristics, some indoor environmental exposures, some allergic manifestations, and subjective symptom reports. Indoor Air Supplement 1994; 2:9–148.

68. Teinjoinsalo J, Jaakola JJ, Seppanen O: The Helsinki Office Study: Air change in mechanically ventilated buildings. Indoor Air 1996;6:111–117.

69. Ten Brinke J, Selvin S, Hodgson AT, et al: Development of new volatile organic compound exposure metrics and their relationship to "sick-building syndrome" symptoms. Indoor Air 1998;8:140-152.

70. Tencati JR, Novey HS: Hypersensitivity angiitis caused by fumes from heat-activated photocopy paper. Ann Intern Med 1983;98:320–322.

71. Tsubota K: Tear dynamics and dry eye. Prog Retin Eye Res 1998;17:565–596.

72. Tsubota K, Nakamori K : Dry eyes and video display terminals.N Engl J Med 1993;328:584.

73. Turiel I, Hollowell CD, Miksch RR: The effects of reduced ventilation on indoor air quality in an office building. Atmos Environ 1983;17:51–64.

74. Wallace LA: Recent field studies of personal and indoor exposures to environmental pollutants. Ann N Y Acad Sci 1992;641:7–16.

75. Wechsler CJ, Shields HC: Production of the hydroxyl radical in indoor air. Environ Sci Technol 1996;30:3250–3258.

76. Wechsler CJ, Shields HC: Indoor ozone/terpene reactions as a source of indoor particles AWWMA meeting 1998; 98–A949

77. Weltermann BM, Hodgson M, Storey E, et al: Hypersensitivity pneumonitis: A sentinel event investigation in a wet building. Am J Ind Med 1998;34:499–505.

78. Wieslander G, Norback D, Nordstrom K, et al: Nasal and ocular symptoms, tear film stability, and biomarkers in nasal lavage, in relation to building dampness and building design in hospitals. Int Arch Occup Environ Health 1999; 72(7):451–461.

79. Willes SR, Bascom R, Fitzgerald TK: Nasal inhalation challenge studies with sidestream tobacco smoke. Arch Environ Health. 1992;47:223–230.

80. Wolkoff Wolkoff P, Clausen G, Fanger PO: Are we measuring the right pollutants? Indoor Air 1997;7:92–106.

81. Woods JE: Cost avoidance and productivity. In Cone J, Hodgson M (eds): Problem Buildings. Occup Med 1989;4:753–770.

82. Wyon D: Sick buildings and the experimental approach. Environ Technol 1992;13:313–322.

83. Zinn WM: Transference phenomena in medical practice: Being whom the patient needs. Ann Intern Med 1990; 113:293–298.

SUSAN P. PROCTOR, DSc

CHEMICAL SENSITIVITY AND GULF WAR VETERANS' ILLNESSES

From the Boston Environmental
  Hazards Center
  and Boston University
Boston, Massachusetts

Reprint requests to:
Susan P. Proctor, DSc
Boston Environmental Hazards
  Center (116B-4)
VA Boston Healthcare System
150 South Huntington Ave.
Boston, MA 02130

Following the Gulf War in 1991, a significant number of the 750,000 veterans from the United States, Great Britain, and Canada began complaining of fatigue, headaches, joint pains, sleep disturbances, cognitive problems, and other somatic symptoms.[7,12] A number of reports have been issued from several "blue ribbon" panels convened to examine these health concerns.[28,29,47,52] Although many of the symptomatic veterans who were clinically evaluated were found to have recognized medical and/or psychological conditions, some did not have symptoms that could be readily explained.[29,50] This has led some veterans groups, clinicians, and media sources to propose the existence of a Gulf War syndrome (GWS) or set of Gulf War syndromes.[25,59]

There have been reports of increased chemical sensitivity in veterans of the Gulf War.[52] Some investigators and veterans question whether the health symptoms reported by returning GW veterans are due to the onset of increased chemical sensitivity triggered by exposures to chemicals during their deployment to the Persian Gulf region in 1990–1991. Other hypotheses that have been put forth to explain GW veterans' illnesses include general stress, traumatic experiences, infectious disease, and specific toxicant exposure.[29,50,52] Some investigators have concluded that GW veterans' illnesses are in fact multiple illnesses with overlapping symptoms due to multiple causes,[18] rather than a unitary syndrome resulting from one specific exposure or event during the Gulf War.

Following is a summary of the current research literature describing GW veterans' health issues as they pertain to chemical sensitivity (CS) and multiple chemical sensitivity (MCS) syndrome. This chapter's orientation is toward research needs for the study and understanding of GW veterans' illnesses. Therefore, the focus is epidemiological research issues, rather than clinical diagnosis and etiology of MCS, both of which are dealt with more substantially elsewhere in this book. Here, the concept that Gulf War syndrome can be explained by MCS is addressed, and arguments for and against this hypothesis are presented.

BACKGROUND: SETTING THE CONTEXT

Since the return of GW military personnel in the spring of 1991, many veterans have reported adverse health symptoms. In registry samples, such as the Department of Veterans Affairs (DVA) GW Registry[46] and the Department of Defense's (DOD) Comprehensive Clinical Evaluation Program[38], and other GW cohort samples[54,67,69] as well as active-duty Air Force veterans,[20] increased rates of various health symptoms have been reported by returning GW veterans. For example, the prevalence of fatigue symptoms is 20–50% in these samples, and problems with concentration have been reported by 14–34%. Furthermore, anecdotal reports have indicated that the complaints appear to persist over time. Additionally, cross-sectional epidemiological studies have noted increased health symptomatology and lower functional status in troops returning from GW deployment as part of Operation Desert Shield/Storm when they are compared to other GW-era veterans, such as nondeployed military personnel,[20,21,24,31,32,64] or to troops deployed to Germany during the same time period.[54,56]

Hypotheses have been raised about increased health concerns in deployed GW veterans, several pointing to specific GW deployment experiences, i.e., service-related environmental exposures, stressful experiences, and exposure to infectious agents.[28,52] Purported Gulf War-service environmental exposures capable of producing these reported symptoms include exposure to the neurotoxicants pyridostigmine bromide (anti-nerve gas pills)[16,34]; nerve agents[23] such as sarin; pesticides[13] and insect repellents[58]; and exposure to products of combustion found in smoke from oil well fires, tent heaters, and burning human wastes.[9,60] It is possible that the Iraqis deployed chemical warfare agents in the Scud missile attacks. Military personnel may also have been exposed to sarin (and other nerve agents) during allied destruction of Iraqi chemical warfare supplies.[33] In addition, several investigations have demonstrated that severe stress can affect physical well-being in veterans.[17,39,68] It has been suggested that the "stress" of exposure to traumatic, wartime events contributes to GW veterans' health symptoms[52] and results in increased health issues characterized by a set of chronic, somatic symptoms (e.g., fatigue, shortness of breath, headaches, sleep disturbances, forgetfulness, and impaired concentration). This hypothesis was supported by examples from prior conflicts.[27]

In this chapter, the term *chemical sensitivity* is used to describe the general phenomenon of feeling ill in response to common chemical exposures such as perfumes, glues, paints, gasoline, or vehicle exhaust. The term *multiple chemical sensitivity* is reserved for the diagnosis of MCS syndrome, based on applying specific case-definition criteria to subjects presenting with somatic symptoms in response to exposure to chemicals at doses below those known to cause harmful effects in the general population.

Several **screening instruments** have been designed that assess chemical sensitivity symptoms and/or their impact on one's lifestyle. These include the Chemical Odor Intolerance Index,[62] Environmental Exposure and Sensitivity Index,[45] a four-item life impact screen by Simon et al.[61] (hereafter referred to as the Simon survey), and a 122-item questionnaire by Kipen and colleagues.[35] For example, in the Simon survey, endorsement of three out of four lifestyle changes was considered to be a specific (although not sensitive) indicator of environmental illness. The four included following a special diet, taking precautions in your home or with home furnishing, wearing particular clothing, or trouble shopping in stores or eating in restaurants because of chemical sensitivity. Other more recent studies have offered additions to the list of lifestyle changes.[6,37] As acknowledged by Szarek et al.,[62] the screening criteria put forth by Simon et al.[61] tend to identify those persons with more severe functional impairments.

Currently, there is no one generally accepted **definition** or set of **diagnostic criteria** for MCS, although several have been proposed and used in research and clinical practice.[2,10,43,48,49] For example, Cullen's research definition of MCS[10] is often applied in clinical settings to make a diagnosis of MCS. The definition is based on symptoms and historical criteria because objective laboratory tests confirming the existence of MCS do not exist. As originally proposed, persons with other definable clinical conditions such as asthma are excluded from the Cullen case definition for MCS, but persons with psychological conditions such as somatization disorder or depression are not excluded.

Another case definition for MCS, proposed by Ashford and Miller,[1] is that a person with MCS is identified by, first, removing the subject from the suspected agents and low-level background chemical exposures (termed the period of *unmasking*) and, second, rechallenging with the agents under controlled environmental conditions. If the person's symptoms clear and then recur, the person is said to have MCS. These researchers stress the need for an environmental medical unit where persons can be removed from everyday exposures in order to accurately measure rates of MCS.

Several surveys have assessed CS and MCS symptoms in general population groups either for comparison to rates observed in MCS patient groups[11] or to examine the general prevalence of MCS syndrome.[3,37,42] The prevalence of CS was 14–66%, depending on the population under study and the assessment protocol used. In an annual telephone survey of randomly selected adults in California assessing a variety of health-related behaviors,[37] 6% (or 253 of 4046 respondents) reported a physician-diagnosed environmental illness or MCS. However, none of these population studies appear to have used a questionnaire instrument that has been validated on persons with clinically diagnosed MCS,[26,35] or articulated how the survey items might correspond with proposed MCS diagnostic criteria. Thus, it is difficult to compare CS prevalence between studies or address the prevalence of MCS in the population groups under study.

FINDINGS: SUMMARY OF STUDIES EXAMINING CS AND MCS IN GULF WAR VETERANS

Similar to what has been observed in review of general population studies of CS and MCS, very few of the studies published or presented to date involving GW veterans have examined CS and/or MCS using the same methodology. Therefore, drawing conclusions about the rates of MCS-like outcomes in GW veteran populations and whether these rates differ from that observed in the general population is difficult. Depending on the population of GW veterans studied and the assessment instruments or criteria used, the rates of CS are 36–86% in DVA patient populations and 0.8–20% in general cohorts of GW veterans. The rates of presumptive MCS, based on a priori MCS case criteria, are 2–6% in studies involving GW veteran cohort samples (Table 1).

TABLE 1. Studies Examining CS and MCS in Gulf War Veterans[†]

Reference	Populations Studied	Instruments Used/ Outcome Assessed	Findings
Bell et al.[4]	DVA outpatients	Telephone survey/CS	• GW-deployed: 63% CS (rate was 86% or 12/14 within those defined as currently feeling ill) GW-era veterans: 41% CS (rate was 57% or 4/7 within those defined as currently feeling ill)
Kipen et al.[36]	Random sample from VA's GW Registry (in 1995)	Mail survey/CS and lifestyle changes	• 36% reported CS • 13.1% report score ≥ 3 & 32.6% report ≥ 2 on Simon survey
Fukuda et al.[20]	Current Active-duty Air Force personnel from four different units (GW deployed and GW-era veterans)	Mail survey/CS	• GW-deployed: 5% CS GW era: 2% CS
Unwin et al.[64]	Stratified, random sample of GW-deployed, Bosnia-deployed, & non-deployed GW-era veterans	Mail survey/CS	* GW-deployed: 0.8% CS Bosnia-deployed: 0.4% CS Non-deployed era: 0.2% CS
Black et al.[6]	Stratified, random sample of GW-deployed and GW-era, non-deployed	Telephone survey/MCS case criteria	* GW-deployed: 5.6% MCS GW-era: 2.6% MCS
Goss Gilroy, Inc.[21]	All Canadian GW-deployed veterans and sample of Canadian Forces who served elsewhere during GW	Mail survey/MCS case criteria	* GW-deployed only: 2.8% MCS (GW-deployed with other conflict history: 2.7%) GW-era only: 0.5% MCS (GW-era with other conflict history: 0.9%)
Proctor et al.[55]	Stratified, random samples of GW veterans from New England (NE) and Louisiana (LA) and comparison group of Germany-deployed GW-era veterans	In-person interview & questionnaire/CS, lifestyle changes, and MCS case criteria	* GW-deployed from NE: 21.1% * GW-deployed from LA: 19.0% Germany-deployed: 2.2% (unadjusted rates) * GW-deployed: 1.2% report ≥ 3 & 2.0% report ≥ 2 on Simon survey Germany deployed: 0% report > 1 * GW-deployed from NE: 2.2% Germany-deployed: 0%

[†] A summary of assessment methods used and results published, in press, and/or presented at the 1999 CDC-sponsored conference entitled The Health Impact of Chemical Exposures during the Gulf War: A Research Planning Conference[8]
CS = chemical sensitivity; MCS = multiple chemical sensitivity; GW = Gulf War
* Rates for GW-deployed veterans

Descriptions of the Different Assessment Methodologies

CHEMICAL SENSITIVITY OR ODOR INTOLERANCE

Bell et al.[4] studied a group of Tucson VA Medical Center outpatients, 24 GW veterans and 17 GW-era veterans. Subjects were asked to complete a telephone survey in which they were queried about ratings of their health and sensitivity to 17 common chemical exposures, both currently and prior to their service. The exposures included perfume, pesticides, drying paint, car exhaust, new carpeting, diesel exhaust, nail polish, gasoline, tobacco smoke, asphalt/tar, paint thinner, hairspray, bleach, natural gas, disinfectants, insect repellent, and chlorinated tap water. GW veterans also were asked about their exposure experiences during the Gulf War. In summary, the rates of CS were higher in GW veterans compared to GW-era veteran patients, with the highest rates reported by veterans indicating they were currently ill.

Miller and Prihoda[44] conducted a case-control study that included a sample of 72 GW veterans, along with two groups of MCS patients, a group of patients with surgical implants, and a group of nonpatient control subjects. Whether the GW veterans studied consisted of persons reporting to be sick is not clear from the article. Each study subject was administered the Environmental Exposure and Sensitivity Inventory (EESI), which provided a continuous score for each of the inventory subscales (Symptom Severity, Chemical Intolerance, Other Intolerance, Life Impact, and Masking Index), and for the EESI overall. Thus, group comparisons were made, but the prevalence rates of CS and lifestyle changes/impacts were not determined. For each of the first four subscales, the control group reported significantly lower scores compared to the four other subject groups. On the mean Masking Index, GW veterans did not differ significantly from controls, but both groups reported significantly higher masking scores (or lower avoidance of regular use of certain medications, caffeine, alcohol, and nicotine) compared with the two MCS groups and the implant group. No adjustment for demographic differences between groups was made when conducting these comparison analyses.

In a recent study by Kipen et al.,[36] a questionnaire was mailed to a randomly selected subsample of 1935 veterans enrolled in the DVA's GW Registry, i.e., GW veterans who have volunteered to participate in a standardized DVA examination protocol. Subjects were asked a general question about whether they considered themselves to be especially sensitive to certain chemicals. They were also asked the four-item Simon survey of lifestyle changes. No comparison population was included in this study.

Subjects in the study by Fukuda et al.[20] of 3723 currently active-duty Air Force personnel (1155 had been GW-deployed) were asked one question about chemical sensitivity in their general list of symptoms. Significantly higher reporting of chemical sensitivity was observed for the GW-deployed group compared to the nondeployed group on this one question.

Unwin et al.[64] used a shortened version of a 122-item screening questionnaire[35] that asked about feelings of ill health when exposed to a variety of common chemical exposures in their study of 3284 GW-deployed, 1815 Bosnia-deployed, and 2408 GW-era veterans from the United Kingdom. However, neither the algorithm used to "score" this questionnaire version nor a description of the subset of the 122 items was provided in the article. The rates of chemical sensitivity were low (< 1%) in all groups and not statistically significantly different from each other after controlling for sociodemographic and lifestyle variables.

MCS CRITERIA-BASED DIAGNOSES

In two related case-control studies of GW veterans recruited from the DVA GW Registry and designed primarily to look at GW veterans with fatiguing illnesses,[15,51] subjects were considered to have a diagnosis of MCS if they reported sensitivity to five of eight chemical odors (pesticides, car exhaust, cologne/aftershave/perfume, new carpet, paint, detergent aisle in grocery store, beauty parlor or barber shop, newly printed newspaper) *or* unusual sensitivity to everyday chemicals *and* endorsed at least two of the four lifestyle changes on the Simon survey. Almost half the veterans who received a diagnosis of chronic fatigue syndrome also had a concurrent diagnosis of MCS.

In a study of a stratified, random sample of Iowa GW- and GW-era veterans,[31] subjects were classified as meeting MCS/idiopathic environmental illness (IEI) criteria if they reported that routine or normal exposure to chemicals caused them to feel ill *and* (1) they were sensitive to at least two in a list of exposures (air pollution; cigarette smoke; vehicle exhaust; copiers or office printing machines; newsprint; pesticides; new buildings; carpeting; organic chemicals, solvents, or paints; perfumes, cosmetics, or hairsprays; or other) *and* (2) they reported symptoms from at least two different categories of symptoms (constitutional, rheumatological, neurological, cardiovascular, gastroenterological, dermatological, pulmonary, or cognitive) *and* (3) the symptoms had led the subject to make a behavioral or lifestyle change in at least one way (wearing a mask, changing lifestyle to minimize exposure, moving to a new home or location, using special vitamins or diets, or using oxygen, antifungals, or neutralizing injections).[5,6] Those deployed to the GW were more likely to meet criteria for MCS/IEI compared to those not deployed (odds ratio = 1.92; 95% confidence interval: 1.22, 3.04).

Similar MCS case criteria was applied in a recent study of Canadian GW veterans,[21] except the lifestyle change criteria were omitted as a requirement for reporting of "symptoms of MCS, without practices to mitigate." As was observed in the Iowa study, those deployed to the GW were more likely to meet criteria for MCS compared to those not deployed (odds ratio = 4.01; 95% confidence interval: 2.43, 6.62).

In a recent study carried out at the Boston Environmental Hazards Center,[55,57] methodology was included to assess CS, lifestyle changes due to chemical sensitivity, and presumptive MCS (based on a set of diagnostic criteria) in stratified, random samples of GW veterans that have been followed longitudinally (from New England and Louisiana) and a comparison group of military personnel deployed to Germany during the time of the GW.[54,70] Chemical sensitivity was assessed from participants' responses a questionnaire. To be designated as having CS, participants met at least one of three criteria. The first criterion required a positive response to at least two of the four Simon survey questions addressing lifestyle changes, representing a modified cut-off score proposed by Simon et al.[61] The second criterion required that participants respond positively to at least two of four questions ascertaining whether food and/or alcohol aversions began or worsened following the Gulf War (e.g., "Does drinking a small amount of alcohol make you feel ill?"). The final criterion required a positive response to feeling ill after exposure to at least two of 12 common odors following the Gulf War. These 12 exposures included new carpeting, insecticides, tobacco smoke, paint thinner, natural gas, perfume/cologne, detergent aisle, hairspray, drying paint, diesel or gas engine exhaust, gasoline, and chlorinated water.

As part of the semi-structured environmental interview administered to each subject in this study, participants were asked to report their dates of deployment, unit assignment, military occupation code, locations in the Gulf (or in Germany), exposures to any hazardous substances while deployed, and current health symptoms. Participants answering in the affirmative to the last two items were systematically queried about the types of substances or exposure scenarios (frequency, duration, intensity, use of personal protective equipment), and about each of their currently reported health symptoms (frequency, duration, intensity, start date for symptom, any days of work lost in past month, initial and/or current triggers of symptom, and course of symptom). Each exposure and health symptom described was coded. Participants who noted a reaction to chemical odors as a symptom trigger were questioned to see if they met a priori research criteria for **presumptive MCS**, based on a modification of Cullen's research criteria.[10] These criteria required that (1) the participant report more than one symptom that began after the Gulf War, (2) these symptoms must involve more than one organ system, and (3) the symptoms must be triggered by low-level exposures to common chemicals. Participants were not excluded for having a concurrent psychiatric diagnosis or for having asthma, but that information was noted. If persons reported symptom(s) on interview that were triggered by low-level exposures to common chemicals but did not fully meet the rest of the criteria, they were categorized as having CS.

The prevalence rates were higher in the GW-deployed groups compared to the Germany-deployed group for both CS and presumptive MCS. However, differences in the rates of presumptive MCS between the GW-deployed and Germany-deployed groups were not significant. Three of the four persons from the New England area, Fort Devens cohort who met criteria for presumptive MCS also met criteria for chronic fatigue syndrome; two reported a diagnosis of asthma; and two also were diagnosed with a psychiatric disorder on clinical interview.[57]

METHODOLOGICAL ISSUES

Although within recent years several epidemiological studies have examined the rates of CS and MCS in GW veteran and comparison populations, a number of research issues need to be addressed to help draw specific conclusions about the prevalence of MCS in GW veterans and examine issues related to etiology, prevention, and treatment strategies within this population.

Based on a critical review of the literature examining CS and MCS in GW veterans, several problem areas are evident. When designing or evaluating future studies, the investigator (and reviewer) should consider a number of specific issues (Table 2) to systematically build on the current state of the science in this topic area.

Use of consistent and/or overlapping definitions of outcome or diagnostic criteria. In the studies described above, none used exactly the same methods of assessing either CS or MCS. Therefore, in most instances, the comparison of

TABLE 2. Research Issues in Studies of CS and MCS in GW Veterans

• Consistent and/or overlapping diagnostic criteria.
• Appropriate and reliable outcome assessment tools.
• Appropriate control or comparison groups to address generalizability of results across studies.
• Assessment of risk factors and comorbid conditions.
• Inclusion of methods to evaluate motivation and other issues such as recall bias that might affect interpretation of self-reported information.
• Assessment of baseline characteristics or changes since GW deployment.
• Concurrent inclusion of standardized health assessment measures.

prevalence rates cannot be direct. Studies by Kipen et al.[36] and Proctor et al.[55] did include the four-item Simon survey to assess the impact of CS on lifestyle, and found significantly different rates (30% vs. 2%, respectively), most likely due to the different GW-deployed cohorts surveyed. Black et al.[5] and Goss Gilroy, Inc.[21] used almost identical criteria for MCS, thus allowing some degree of comparison across studies.

Depending on study design, the use of several different assessment methods (such as was done in the study by Proctor and colleagues[55]) is recommended. This "tiered" assessment approach, i.e., including diagnostic criteria as well as validated scales to assess symptomatology, has been advocated by Fukuda et al.[19] for assessing chronic fatigue syndrome.

Use of appropriate, reliable assessment tools. Regardless of the mode of assessment (e.g., mail questionnaire, telephone survey, in-person interview and/or clinical evaluation), it would be useful to include assessment measures that have been tested or validated in clinical patient populations diagnosed with MCS using a priori criteria. Three such screening questionnaires that assess CS for which there is some supportive validation information are those developed by Kipen et al.,[35] Szarek et al.,[62] and Miller and Prihoda.[45] Also, a shortened version of Kipen and colleagues' 122-item questionnaire has been proposed by Hu et al.[26] as an instrument to discriminate between subjects with and without MCS symptomatology.

Inclusion of appropriate comparison groups to address the generalizability of results. For assessing prevalence rates, it is important to include a control or comparison group, particularly if the study group is not representative of the general GW-deployed population. For example, when examining CS and/or MCS in treatment-seeking GW veterans, it is advisable to include a group of treatment-seeking GW-era veterans for comparison, as was done by Bell and colleagues.[4]

Assessment of risk factors and comorbid conditions. Research is needed to explore the relationship between MCS syndromes and other medical and psychiatric conditions. Exploring such relationships may provide some clues as to the underlying etiology of MCS, as well as help in identifying factors that may confound its detection and treatment.

Within the studies of GW veterans described above, some identified risk factors for CS or MCS included being female and African-American[36]; rank and income level[21]; age, branch of service, current psychiatric status, and being on disability compensation[5,6]; and exposure to certain self-reported GW-related exposures such as pesticides.[4]

Inclusion of methods to evaluate motivation and other issues such as recall bias that might affect interpretation of self-reported information. Although self-reported information about symptoms and lifestyle changes is currently the most appropriate and reliable for assessing CS and MCS, additional measures should be included in the study design or analysis phase to allow an evaluation of *recall bias* or *motivation levels*. For example, a surrogate measure for recall bias was calculated in one study by examining the difference in reported GW combat exposure assessed 8 years apart. Wolfe et al.[71] controlled for this variable in multivariate regression analyses performed to predict the risk of multisymptom illness (as defined by Fukuda et al.[20]) in a cross-sectional study of the prospectively followed Devens cohort of GW veterans. Other methods include conducting a test-retest reliability assessment of subject responses, as was done in studies by the Iowa Persian Gulf Study Group[31] and the Portland Environmental Hazards Center,[40,41] or the addition of a test of motivation to the study protocol (such as the Test of Memory Malingering[63]).

Assessment of baseline characteristics or changes since GW deployment. The Gulf War occurred approximately 10 years ago; thus, numerous intervening life events may have occurred to influence current health status. When examining current health in relationship to GW events or experiences, the impacts of intervening events should be addressed when possible. Longitudinal cohort studies begun shortly after the GW, rather than currently initiated retrospective studies, may be better able to address these impacts.

Concurrent inclusion of standardized health assessment measures. Most of the GW population studies described above[5,15,20,21,56,57,64] have included the Medical Outcomes Study 36-item Short Form,[65,66] a well-validated instrument for measurement of functional status. Extensive norms from U.S. populations and patients with various medical conditions are available for this scale, allowing better examination of the impact of health/medical outcomes on functional status. Black et al.[5] found that more functional impairment was observed in persons meeting MCS case criteria than those not meeting the criteria. Mean or median levels also can be compared to levels observed in population groups with other medical conditions.

SUMMARY

Depending on the population of GW veterans studied and the assessment instruments or criteria used, the rates of CS range from 36–86% in DVA populations of GW veteran patients, and between 0.8–20% in general cohort studies of GW veterans. The rates of presumptive MCS, based on varying a priori MCS case criteria, range from 2–6% in studies involving GW veteran cohort samples. In most studies, these rates are higher than those observed in nondeployed comparison groups. However, adjustment for demographic and lifestyle variables between groups was not always made.

When making across-study comparisons of the rates of CS and MCS observed in general GW veteran cohort studies to rates observed in general population studies, the rates observed in GW veterans are not substantially higher. As expressed above, drawing conclusions is difficult as different assessment methodologies were used in these various studies.

Future Directions

Further research to evaluate the relationship between CS and MCS in GW veterans needs to proceed on two fronts: (1) continue targeted study of GW veterans' health issues in general, and (2) focus on the basic epidemiology of CS and MCS to expand our knowledge about these conditions in the general population. In both instances, attention to the above-identified methodological issues is recommended. Several recent research directives[30,53] and commissioned reviews[22] have suggested similar research directions in this area. Specifically, prospective studies and longitudinal analyses of the health status of GW veterans and other military personnel as they proceed through future pre- and post-deployment periods, and/or studies of the incidence of CS and MCS within the general population and within cohorts of susceptible individuals, are needed.

CONTROVERSY

Is Gulf War syndrome the same thing as multiple chemical sensitivity syndrome? In other words, can GW veterans' health concerns be explained by heightened sensitivity to low-level chemical exposures triggered by exposures to chemicals during the Gulf War?

For: The studies summarized here indicate that higher rates of CS and MCS are observed in GW-deployed military personnel compared to nondeployed GW-era veterans, suggesting that deployment to the GW may be a predictor or initiating factor for heightened chemical sensitivity. The persistence of health symptoms reported by GW veterans over the 9 years since the end of the Gulf War supports the idea that low-level exposures to everyday chemicals operate as reoccurring triggers, which can be accounted for by a process in which the "smells of war" are linked to physiological reactions (as hypothesized by Fergusson and Cassaday[14]).

Against: The rates of CS/MCS in GW veterans are lower than the rates of health symptom complaints in these veterans. It appears likely that GW veterans' illnesses are not all caused by the same mechanism.

Opinion: Given the current state of knowledge about GW veterans' health problems or illnesses and about CS and MCS in this population, it is this author's opinion that MCS and a unitary GWS are *not* the same entity. Borrowing from the paradigms put forth by Cullen to graphically depict the distinctions between MCS and other "environmental" disorders,[10] this author proposes that there is some overlap between GW veterans with health complaints and GW veterans with MCS (Fig. 1).

The proportion of GW veterans included in the overlap is difficult to determine given the current literature. In the study by Bell and colleagues[4] involving GW veteran VA outpatients, 86% or 12/14 of those who rated themselves as currently ill also reported symptoms of CS. In contrast, results from a recent assessment of GW veterans (Devens cohort) conducted by Wolfe and colleagues (personal communication; analyses in progress), indicate that 22% or 170/780 of GW veterans who met the CDC case definition for multisymptom illness (as put forth by Fukuda et al.[20]) also met criteria for MCS using the validated screening questionnaire proposed by Hu et al.[26]

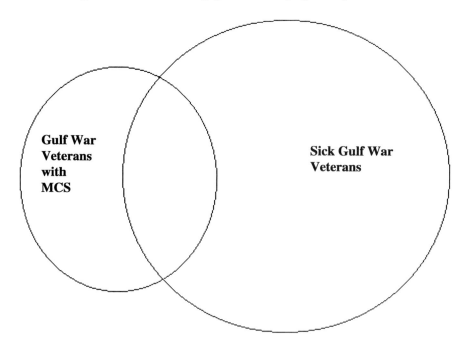

FIGURE 1. Venn diagram of relationship between MCS and ill GW veterans.

At this point in time, additional research is needed to more definitely answer the question about whether GW veterans' health concerns are explained by heightened sensitivity to low-level chemical exposures triggered by exposures to chemicals during the Gulf War.

ACKNOWLEDGEMENTS

The author is currently supported by funding from the Department of Veterans Affairs (DVA) Office of Research and Development (Boston Environmental Hazards Center), Centers for Disease Control and Prevention (U50/CCU114464-03), and Department of Defense (#DAMD17-00-1-0064; #DAMD17-00-1-0063). Additional earlier funding support was provided by the DVA Mental Health Strategic Healthcare Group to the National Center for PTSD and by the Department of Defense (#DAMD17-95-1-5047; #DAMD17-96-1-6043).

The author would like to thank Roberta F. White, PhD and Howard Hu, MD, ScD for their comments on an earlier version of this manuscript, and Erik Rosenman, BA and Kristin Heaton, MS for their assistance in the manuscript preparation. In addition, the author acknowledges Jessica Wolfe, PhD and Chaplain William Mark for their foresight and efforts on behalf of the Ft. Devens Operation Desert Storm cohort.

REFERENCES
1. Ashford N, Miller C: Chemical Exposures: Low Levels and High Stakes, 2nd ed. New York, Van Nostrand Reinhold, 1998.
2. Bartha L, Baumzweiger W, Buscher DS, et al.: Multiple chemical sensitivity: A 1999 consensus. Arch Environ Health 54(3):147–149, 1999.
3. Bell IR: Self-reported illness from chemical odors in young adults without clinical syndromes or occupational exposures. Arch Environ Health 48(1):6–13, 1993.
4. Bell IR, Warg-Damiani L, Baldwin CM,et al: Self-reported chemical sensitivity and wartime chemical exposures in Gulf War veterans with and without decreased global health ratings. Mil Med 163(11):725–732, 1998.
5. Black DW, Doebbeling BN, Voelker MD, et al.: Quality of life and health-services utilization in a population-based sample of military personnel reporting multiple chemical sensitivities. J Occup Environ Med 41(10):928–933, 1999.
6. Black DW, Doebbeling BN, Voelker MD, et al: Multiple chemical sensitivity syndrome: Symptom prevalence and risk factors in a military population. Arch Intern Med 160:1169–1176, 2000.
7. Centers for Disease Control and Prevention: Unexplained illness among Persian Gulf War veterans in an Air National Guard unit: Preliminary report- August 1990-March 1995. MMWR Morbid Mortal Weekly Report 44:443–447, 1995 (also appears as Kizer KW, Joseph S, Moll M, Rankin JT: Unexplained illness among Persian Gulf War veterans in an Air National Guard unit. JAMA 274:16–17, 1995).
8. Centers for Disease Control and Prevention: Conference Proceedings—The Health Impact of Chemical Exposures During the Gulf War: A Research Planning Conference. Atlanta, 1999. Conference transcript can be found at http://www.cdc.gov/nceh/meetings/1999/gulfwar/
9. Costa DL, Amdur MO: Air pollution. In Klaassen CD, Amdur MO, Doull J (eds): Casarett & Doull's Toxicology: The Basic Science of Poisons, 5th ed. New York, McGraw-Hill Health Professions Division, 1996, pp 857–882.
10. Cullen MR: The worker with multiple chemical sensitivities: An overview. Occup Med 2(4):655–661, 1987.
11. Davidoff AL, Keyl PM: Symptoms and health status in individuals with multiple chemical sensitivities syndrome from four reported sensitizing exposures and a general population comparison group. Arch Environ Health 51:201–213, 1996.
12. DeFraites RF, Wanat ER, Norwood AE, et al: Investigation of a Suspected Outbreak of an Unknown Disease among Veterans of Operation Desert Shield/Storm, 123rd Army Reserve Command, Fort Benjamin, Harrison, IN. Washington, DC, Walter Reed Army Institute of Research, 1992.
13. Ecobichon DJ: Toxic effects of pesticides. In Klaassen CD, Amdur MO, Doull J (eds): Casarett & Doull's Toxicology: The Basic Science of Poisons, 5th ed. New York, McGraw-Hill Health Professions Division, 1996, pp 643–689.
14. Ferguson E, Cassaday HJ: The Gulf War and illness by association. Br J Psychol 90:459–475, 1999.
15. Fiedler N, Lange G, Tiersky L, et al: Stressors, personality traits, and coping of Gulf War veterans with chronic fatigue. J Psychsom Res (in press) 2000.

16. Friedman A, Kaufer D, Shemer J, et al: Pyridostigmine brain penetration under stress enhances neuronal excitability and induces early immediate transcriptional response. Nature Med 2:1383–1385, 1996.
17. Friedman MJ, Schnurr PP: The relationship between trauma, post-traumatic stress disorder, and physical health. In Friedman MJ, Charney DS, Deutch AY (eds): Neurobiological and Clinical Consequences of Stress: From Normal Adaptation to Post-Traumatic Stress Disorder. Philadelphia, Lippincott-Raven, 1995, pp 507–524.
18. Frost SD: Gulf War syndrome: Proposed causes. Cleveland Clinic J Med 67:17–20, 2000.
19. Fukuda K, Straus SE, Hickie I, et al. and the International Chronic Fatigue Syndrome Study Group: The chronic fatigue syndrome: A comprehensive approach to its definition and study. Ann Intern Med 121:953–959, 1994.
20. Fukuda K, Nisenbaum R, Stewart G, et al: Chronic multisymptom illness affecting Air Force veterans of the Gulf War. JAMA 280(11):981–988, 1998.
21. Goss Gilroy, Inc.: Health Study of Canadian Forces Personnel Involved in the 1991 Conflict in the Persian Gulf. 1998. Report can be found at http://www.dnd.ca/menu/press/Reports/Health/health_study_eng_1.htm
22. Graveling RA, Pilkington A, George JPK, et al: A review of multiple chemical sensitivity. Occup Environ Med 56:73–85, 1999.
23. Gunderson CH, Lehmann CR, Sidell FR, Jabbari B: Nerve agents: A review. Neurology 42:946–950, 1992.
24. Haley RW, Hom J, Roland PS, et al: Evaluation of neurologic function in Gulf War veterans: A blinded case-control study. JAMA 277:223–230, 1997.
25. Haley RW, Kurt TL, Hom J: Is there a Gulf War syndrome? Searching for syndromes by factor analysis of symptoms. JAMA 277:215–222, 1997.
26. Hu H, Stern A, Rotnitzky A, et al: Development of a brief questionnaire for screening for multiple chemical sensitivity syndrome. Toxicol Indust Health 15:582–588, 1999.
27. Hyams KC, Wignall FS, Roswell R: War syndromes and their evaluation: From the U.S. Civil War to the Persian Gulf War. Ann Intern Med 125:398–405, 1996.
28. Institute of Medicine: Health Consequences of Service During the Persian Gulf War: Initial Findings and Recommendations for Immediate Action. Washington, DC, National Academy Press, 1995.
29. Institute of Medicine: Evaluation of the Department of Defense Persian Gulf Comprehensive Clinical Evaluation Program. Division of Health Promotion and Disease Prevention. Washington, DC, National Academy Press, 1996.
30. Institute Of Medicine: Gulf War Veterans: Measuring Health. Washington, DC, National Academy Press, 1999.
31. Iowa Persian Gulf Study Group: Self-reported illness and health status among Gulf War veterans: A population-based study. JAMA 277(3):238–245, 1997.
32. Ishoy T, Guldager B, Appleyard M, et al: State of health after deployment in the Persian Gulf. Danish Medical Bulletin 46(5):416–419, 1999 (English); Ugeskr Laeger 161(39):5423–5328, 1999.
33. Joseph S: Testimony to the Subcommittee on Human Resources and Intergovernmental Relations, Committee on Government Reform and Oversight, U.S. House of Representatives, June 25, 1996.
34. Keeler JR, Hurst CG, Dunn MA: Pyridostigmine used as a nerve agent pretreatment under wartime conditions. JAMA 266: 693–695, 1991.
35. Kipen HM, Hallman W, Kelly-McNeil K, Fiedler N: Measuring chemical sensitivity prevalence: A questionnaire for population studies. Am J Public Health 85:574–577, 1994.
36. Kipen HM, Hallman W, Kang H, Fiedler N, Natelson BH: Prevalence of chronic fatigue and chemical sensitivities in Gulf Registry veterans. Arch Environ Health 54(5):313–318, 1999.
37. Kreutzer R, Neutra RR, Lashuay N: Prevalence of people reporting sensitivities to chemicals in a population-based survey. Am J Epidemiol 150(1):1–12, 1999.
38. Kroenke K, Koslow P, Roy M: Symptoms in 18,495 Persian Gulf War veterans. J Occup Environ Med 40:520–528, 1998.
39. Kulka RA, Schlenger WE, Fairbank JA: Trauma and the Vietnam War Generation. New York, Brunner/Mazel, 1990.
40. McCauley LA, Joos SK, Spencer PS, et al. and members of the Portland Environmental Hazards Research Center: Strategies to assess validity of self-reported exposures during the Persian Gulf War. Environ Res Section A 81:195–205, 1999.
41. McCauley LA, Joos SK, Lasarev M, et al: Gulf War unexplained illnesses: Persistence and unexplained nature of self-reported symptoms. Environ Res Section A 81:215–223, 1999.
42. Meggs WJ, Dunn KA, Bloch RM, et al: Prevalence and nature of allergy and chemical sensitivity in a general population. Arch Environ Health 51:275–282, 1996.
43. Miller CS: Toxicant-induced loss of tolerance: An emerging theory of disease? Environ Health Perspect 105(suppl 2):445–453, 1997.

44. Miller CS, Prihoda TJ: A controlled comparison of symptoms and chemical intolerances reported by Gulf War veterans, implant recipients, and persons with multiple chemical sensitivity. Toxicol Ind Health 15:386–397, 1999.
45. Miller CS, Prihoda TJ: The Environmental Exposure and Sensitivity Inventory: A standardized approach for measuring chemical intolerances for research and clinical applications. Toxicol Ind Health 15:370–385, 1999.
46. Murphy FM, Kang H, Dalager NA, et al.: The health status of Gulf War veterans: Lessons learned from the Department of Veterans Affairs Health Registry. Mil Med 164(5):327–331, 1999.
47. National Institutes of Health Technology Assessment Workshop Panel: The Persian Gulf experience and health. JAMA 272:391–396, 1994.
48. National Research Council (NRC): Multiple Chemical Sensitivities: Addendum to Biologic Markers in Immunotoxicology. Washington, DC, National Academy Press, 1992.
49. Nethercott JR, Davidoff LL, Curbow B, Abbey H: Multiple chemical sensitivities syndrome: Toward a working case definition. Arch Environ Health 48:19–26, 1993.
50. Persian Gulf Veterans Coordinating Board: Unexplained illnesses among Desert Storm veterans. Arch Intern Med 155:262–268, 1995.
51. Pollet C, Natelson BH, Lange G, et al: Medical evaluation of Persian Gulf veterans with fatigue and/or chemical sensitivity. J Med 29:101–113, 1998.
52. Presidential Advisory Committee on Gulf War Veterans' Illnesses (PAC Report): Final Report. Washington DC, U.S. Government Printing Office, 1996.
53. Presidential Review Directive 5: A National Obligation: Planning for Health Preparedness for and Readjustment of the Military, Veterans, and their Families after Future Deployment. Executive Office of the President; Office of Science and Technology Policy. Released on November 11, 1998 on Internet at http://www1.whitehouse.gov/WH/EOP/OSTP/NSTC/html/directive5.html.
54. Proctor SP, Heeren T, White RF, et al.: Health status of Persian Gulf War veterans: Self-reported symptoms, environmental exposures, and the effect of stress. Int J Epidemiol 27:1000–1010, 1998.
55. Proctor SP, Wolfe J, White RF: Boston Environmental Hazards Center: Research on Multiple Chemical Sensitivity and Gulf War Veterans. Presented at the CDC-sponsored conference The Health Impact of Chemical Exposures During the Gulf War: A Research Planning Conference. Atlanta, 1999. Conference transcript can be found at http://www.cdc.gov/nceh/meetings/1999/gulfwar/
56. Proctor SP, Harley R, Wolfe J, et al: Health-related quality of life in Gulf War veterans. Submitted.
57. Proctor SP, Heaton KJ, White RF, Wolfe J: Chemical sensitivity and chronic fatigue in Gulf War veterans: A brief report. Submitted.
58. Robbins PJ, Cherniack MG: Review of the biodistribution and toxicity of the insect repellent N, N-diethyl-m-toluamide (DEET). J Toxicol Environ Health 18:503–525, 1986.
59. Robinson A: Veterans worry that unexplained medical problems a legacy of service during Gulf War. Can Med Assoc J 152:944–947, 1995.
60. Shusterman DJ: Clinical smoke inhalation injury: Systemic effects. Occup Med 8(3):469–503, 1993.
61. Simon GE, Katon WJ, Sparks PJ: Allergic to life: Psychological factors in environmental illness. Am J Psychiatry 147:901–906, 1990.
62. Szarek MJ, Bell IR, Schwartz GE: Validation of a brief screening measures of environmental chemical sensitivity: The Chemical Odor Intolerance Index. J Environ Psychol 17:345–351, 1997.
63. Tombaugh T: Test of Memory Malingering. North Tonawanda, NY, Multi-Health Systems, Inc., 1996.
64. Unwin C, Blatchley N, Coker W, et al: Health of UK servicemen who served in the Persian Gulf War. Lancet 353:169–178, 1999.
65. Ware J: SF36 Health Survey: Manual and Interpretation Guide. Boston, The Health Institute, 1993.
66. Ware J: SF36 Physical and Mental Health Summary Scales: A User's Manual. Boston, The Health Institute, 1994.
67. Wolfe J, Brown P, Kelly JM: Reassessing war stress: Exposure and the Persian Gulf War. J Social Issues 49(4):15–31, 1993.
68. Wolfe J, Schnurr PP, Brown PJ, Furey J: PTSD and war-zone exposure as correlates of perceived health in female Vietnam veterans. J Consult Clin Psychol 162:1235–1240, 1994.
69. Wolfe J, Proctor SP, Davis J, Borgos M, Friedman M: Health symptoms reported by Persian Gulf War veterans two years after their return. Am J Ind Med 33:104–113, 1998.
70. Wolfe J, Proctor SP, Erickson D, et al.: Relationship of psychiatric status to Gulf War veterans' health problems. Psychosom Med 61:532–540, 1999.
71. Wolfe J, Erickson D, Proctor SP, et al: Risk factors for the development of multisymptom illness in U.S. veterans of the Gulf War: Ft. Devens ODS Reunion Cohort Study. Submitted.

PATRICIA J. SPARKS, MD, MPH

DIAGNOSTIC EVALUATION AND TREATMENT OF THE PATIENT PRESENTING WITH IDIOPATHIC ENVIRONMENTAL INTOLERANCE

From Private Consulting Practice
Occupational and Environmental
  Medicine and Clinical Toxicology
Mercer Island, Washington

Reprint requests to:
Patricia J. Sparks, MD, MPH
Occupational and Environmental
  Medicine and Clinical Toxicology
7683 SE 27th Street, PMB #291
Mercer Island, WA 98040

Understanding the phenomenon of idiopathic environmental intolerance (IEI) requires evaluation of pathophysiologic, psychological, and social factors using the biopsychosocial model of illness. The comprehensive biopsychosocial model[9] is a systems approach that conceptualizes an intimate mind-body connection: physical diseases have psychological and social correlates, and psychological illnesses have physical correlates. *Illness should not be regarded as less "real" because of the possibility that psychogenic mechanisms may play a major role in causation for many sufferers. The IEI patient's distress should never be dismissed with a statement that it is "all in the head."*

Clinicians with different views about the pathogenesis of IEI still may agree on clinical management programs aimed at symptom control and improved functional ability rather than "cure" of IEI.[28]

GENERAL PRINCIPLES

Before discussing further the clinical evaluation of the patient presenting with IEI, let us review the basic principles of assessing causal relationship between the any patient's illness and specific chemical exposures. Methods for investigating causal relationships between agents and illness exist and are well described in the scientific literature.[14] A conclusion about cause and effect relationship must be supported by scientific evidence such that the relationship has been demonstrated and, therefore, can occur. The causal connection between a disorder and a toxic substance must be established as a general principle before it can be established in an individual. Next, the exposure to the alleged causal agent has to be established, and the dosage (amount and duration of exposure) has to have been sufficient to cause the disease.

In determining causal relationship of exposure and disease in any individual, determine the following:
- Does the patient have a recognizable disease? What is the diagnosis?
- Can the agent(s) of concern produce this disorder?
- Are there substantial and properly relevant animal data?
- Is there human evidence? Are there well-controlled epidemiologic data, and are there confirmatory human toxicological data?
- Did the exposure cause the disorders in this case?
- Have other causes been properly considered and ruled out in the differential diagnosis?
- Has the exposure been confirmed?
- Was the dose sufficient, considering the concentration and duration, to produce the condition?
- Was the clinical pattern expected from that causal agent?
- Are there objective manifestations of disease consistent with exposure?
- Were the temporal relationship and latency periods appropriate?

Two types of scientific knowledge are essential in evaluating claims of injury from chemical exposure. One is the **confirmation of exposure** and the other is some **indication of dose**. Occupational and environmental exposures to potentially hazardous substances are graded in terms of duration and intensity.

Millions of people in this country are exposed to various chemical substances in the home and workplace every day. They are not all at risk for developing ailments arising from exposure to those chemicals. Even when causal relationship between a specific chemical exposure and disease has been established with consistent epidemiologic and toxicologic data, the risks associated with a particular exposure are determined by the extent and duration of exposure, not the mere fact of exposure. Thus, the fact of an exposure, taken alone, is irrelevant if taken out of context, and especially if taken out of the context of dose-response. The potential health impact of that exposure is dependent on the nature of the chemical, it's specific toxicology, the amount of exposure, the duration, and the route of absorption. The fact that a chemical may be capable of producing an effect, does not mean that any contact at all with the chemical produces the effect.

The physician evaluating a patient with possible chemically related illness must make a judgment about the extent of exposure to a chemical substance or mixture and the capability of the chemical exposure to cause the specific health problems observed in the patient based on the medical/toxicologic/epidemiologic literature. Additionally, he or she must rule out other common conditions with similar complaints in the differential diagnosis. When hearing hoofbeats, the physician should first look for horses rather than zebras.

DIAGNOSTIC EVALUATION

The History and Physical Examination

The keys to diagnosis and clinical management of the individual presenting with suspected or previously diagnosed IEI include a detailed exposure history, as well as a comprehensive medical and psychosocial evaluation of the patient[28] (Table 1).

TABLE 1.   Diagnostic Evaluation for IEI

History
  Detailed exposure history (workplace and other environmental exposures)
  Industrial hygiene data (Material Safety Data Sheets, results of exposure monitoring, etc.)
  Current and past medical illnesses, and results of previous diagnostic work-ups and treatments
  Review of prior medical records
Physical Examination
  Rule out other illnesses in the differential diagnosis
Consultation
  Occupational and environmental medicine specialist
  Psychiatrist
  Other specialists as appropriate to rule out other medical conditions in the differential diagnosis
Other
  Symptom diary
  Short-term removal from exposure

From Sparks PJ, Daniell W, Black DW, et al: Multiple chemical sensitivity syndrome: A clinical perspective. II. Evaluation, diagnostic testing, treatment, and social considerations. J Occup Med 36(7):731–737, 1994; with permission.

It is critical to rule out the presence of a physical disease caused by defined occupational or environmental factors. A *pitfall to avoid* is to inappropriately diagnose patients with well-defined toxic or allergic disease or irritant injury, such as asthma, solvent intoxication, or sinusitis, as having IEI, thus failing to provide appropriate treatment. There also may be some overlap of these conditions and IEI syndrome.

The clinical evaluation of IEI is challenging for the occupational and environmental physician specialist with formal training and experience in exposure assessment and clinical toxicology. Therefore, it may be extremely difficult for the primary care physician, who usually is not trained to evaluate the clinical significance of the patient's exposure history. In most cases, consultation with a physician who is board-certified in occupational and environmental medicine or industrial toxicology should be obtained. The evaluation of a patient presenting with IEI may take several hours, and it is necessary to allot sufficient time.

Obtain industrial hygiene data regarding the patient's exposures whenever possible. If the exposure occurred in the workplace, procure the relevant Material Safety Data Sheets from the patient or employer. Many chemicals are well-established potential causes of the symptoms that IEI patients describe (e.g., toluene diisocyanate and chest tightness, or headache and nausea from exposure to lead or organic solvents). Clearly, it is the physician's job to *estimate the dose* of environmental exposure, and to determine the probability that an individual patient's symptoms are due to a known toxic or irritant effect of exposure.

Some clinicians have suggested having the patient keep a symptom diary throughout the day, along with information regarding activities and environmental exposures. If, however, cultural and physician-shaped belief systems or misdiagnosed psychiatric or physical illness is operative, the patient's perception of the relationship between symptoms and chemical exposures—rather than other potential psychological stressors, for example—may be reinforced. Thus this approach probably is not appropriate for many IEI patients, and there is a fine line between urging the patient to pay attention to the effect of various environmental exposures on their symptoms and promoting symptom attribution by suggestion.

It is essential that the physician rule out other nonenvironmental illness or disease in the differential diagnosis. Take a detailed medical history regarding current and past illnesses, previous diagnostic evaluations and treatments, and a possible historical pattern of many unexplained physical symptoms with onset early in adulthood or frequent utilization of medical care. Access to and thorough review of prior medical and psychiatric records are particularly important. Physical examination and laboratory evaluation should be sufficiently comprehensive to establish or rule out all other occupational and nonoccupational disease conditions in the differential diagnosis.

Psychiatric evaluation of the individual diagnosed with IEI may be appropriate, given the high prevalence of coexisting or preexisting psychiatric disorders in these patients. Unfortunately, most patients given a diagnosis of IEI resist the idea that psychological factors may play any etiologic role at all in their distress; however, this resistance should not be interpreted to mean that the patient has a primary psychiatric illness. The adamant rejection of psychological factors in symptom formation and expression by IEI patients is a challenge for the physician, but the important role of psychological stress in symptom severity should be discussed.

Diagnostic Testing in IEI

Since there is no established and widely available test to use to diagnose IEI, the physician must be extremely cautious about excessive or inappropriate testing or the misinterpretation of such tests. Such actions may merely reinforce a detrimental pattern of illness behavior.[28]

Diagnostic testing in patients expressing symptoms of IEI is necessary primarily to rule out the presence of other environmental or nonenvironmental illness or treatable disease conditions in the differential diagnosis (Table 2). For example, if the patient has prominent respiratory tract complaints, appropriate pulmonary function tests are needed, as a minimum, to rule out the presence of reactive airway disease. Biological monitoring might be used in some cases to assess exposure to specific chemical substances when there is known to be good correlation of the specific exposure with measured blood or urine levels and health effect (e.g., heavy metals). However, results of diagnostic tests should not be presumed to explain multiorgan symptoms. For example, if pulmonary function tests show airway reactivity,

TABLE 2.   Diagnostic Testing for IEI

- No established diagnostic test for IEI
- Done primarily to rule out other illnesses in the differential diagnosis
- Results of test should not be presumed to explain multiorgan symptoms

The following tests currently are *not* validated for clinical use to confirm the diagnosis of IEI:
  Environmental challenge testing (uncontrolled, unblinded)
  Quantitative electroencephalography
  Brain electrical activity mapping
  Evoked potentials (brainstem, visual, sensory)
  Position emission tomography scan
  Single photon emission computed tomography scan
  Immunologic testing
  Measurements of trace concentrations of volatile organic compounds or pesticides in blood
    (parts per billion)
  Neuropsychologic testing
  Blood enzyme tests for porphyrias

From Sparks PJ, Daniell W, Black DW, et al: Multiple chemical sensitivity syndrome: A clinical perspective. II. Evaluation, diagnostic testing, treatment, and social considerations. J Occup Med 36(7):731–737, 1994; with permission.

this does not explain central nervous system, gastrointestinal, dermal, visual, or other organ system complaints.

Also, subtle variations in physiologic testing may be hard to distinguish from normal variability in a heterogeneous population, and caution is necessary so as not to overinterpret results as an explanation for the patient's symptoms. The patient should be informed that normal test results do not indicate that insufficient testing was done, but rather that evidence of organ system damage was not present.[35]

In some patients, hyperventilation may play a significant role in their symptoms. Observation of breathing rate and pattern, chemistry screening for hypophosphatemia, or measurement of arterial blood gases may be indicated.[20]

Definitive research on controlled **challenge procedures** is necessary before they can be recommended as useful tools for diagnosis.[29,30] The clinical use of environmental challenge units for diagnosing IEI remains controversial. The problems with this approach are: (1) we usually do not know the actual level of environmental exposure causing symptoms, (2) testing of substances having distinct odors or irritant properties cannot be done in a blinded fashion, and (3) proper controls and objective measures of response that are relevant to the patient's symptoms are unavailable. Successfully blinded chemical challenges have reportedly resulted in both high false-positive and false-negative rates of response.

Quantitative EEG (QEEG), brain electrical activity mapping (BEAM), evoked potentials, and positron emission tomography (PET) and single photon emission computed tomography (SPECT) scans, which measure regional blood flow or brain metabolic function, have been misapplied in an effort to provide "objective findings" for patients with IEI. Any technique for investigating the CNS effects of low-level exposure to chemical substances should take place only in a research setting with proper controls to validate its clinical use as a diagnostic tool to confirm the presence of IEI.[23,27,34]

A recent controlled epidemiologic study of use of SPECT brain imaging in IEI and chronic fatigue syndrome (CFS) patients[15] used both computerized quantitative methods and qualitative visual methods on all study participants. The study demonstrated nonspecific differences in global perfusion and in the ventricular and anterior cingulate regions of the brain in IEI patients compared to normal and CFS patients using the quantitative technique. The findings could not conclusively distinguish the SPECT findings of IEI cases from patients with anxiety, depression, or obsessive-compulsive disorders. Unfortunately, there is no diagnostic gold standard or tissue pathology to validate findings in IEI patients. The study used a computerized or quantitative method to develop a discriminant function for distinguishing IEI cases from controls, and few differences could be distinguished by the visual methods of analysis used in most laboratories (in this study the specificity by the visual image identification method was only 58%). SPECT imaging is not useful in confirming a diagnosis of IEI at this time.[15,34]

At present, no form of **immunological testing** has been shown to be diagnostic of either exposure to specific chemicals or illness due to exposure in patients with IEI.[24,26,28,33] For example, low titers of antibodies to formaldehyde have not been correlated either with exposure or with disease due to exposure to formaldehyde. Non-traditional tests, such as provocation-neutralization, show no correlation with exposure or disease resulting from specific chemicals,[6,17] and cannot be justified because of lack of evidence of symptom provocation by sub-neutralizing concentrations.

A more recent study of immunologic parameters in IEI patients compared to controls[22] did not reliably distinguish IEI patients from controls such that it could be concluded that any immunologic parameters might be useful in diagnosis.

Some commercial laboratories offer measurements of part per billion concentrations of various organic solvents or other exogenous chemicals in blood. Often the chemicals are reported to be present at concentrations in the range of error noise of mass spectrometer analysis and have no clinical relevance. Unfortunately, some physicians have misinterpreted such measures as evidence of unusual chemical exposure and/or toxicity or as an explanation for the symptoms of IEI. Clinical misuse and misinterpretation of such testing is to be avoided.

Neuropsychological testing is dependent on patient cooperation and might be useful to rule out other conditions in the differential diagnosis, but currently does not reveal consistent or specific findings in IEI patients that may be used for diagnosis of this condition.[5]

Finally, **blood enzyme assays** (corproporphyrin oxidase, for example), or slight increases in urinary coproporphyrin excretion, have been used inappropriately to diagnose various porphyrias or "porphyrinopathies" in IEI. Such testing does not confirm the diagnosis of porphyria in these patients; the enzyme assays have numerous limitations; and there is no scientific evidence supporting a causal link between any of the porphyrias and IEI.[8,13]

Reinforcement of illness behavior by unjustifiably giving a patient the diagnosis of a disease due to toxic, immunological, metabolic or neurological mechanisms based on diagnostic testing that is clinically unsubstantiated or invalid may actually perpetuate illness, prolong disability, and delay effective therapy.

TREATMENT

Even if the etiologies of the symptoms in patients diagnosed with IEI are controversial and unknown in most patients, these individuals still can be helped with their symptoms (Table 3). A nonjudgmental approach to evaluation and treatment, based on the assumption that the patient's symptoms are "real" and distressing regardless of the presence or absence of observable organic pathology, is suggested.[12,28] *The physician may affirm the illness experience without affirming the attribution for it.* The goal of therapy is **control of symptoms**, and success is not dependent on a specific organic diagnosis or etiology, but rather on the patient's acquisition of skills for coping with the illness' impact on daily life and improved understanding of the role of stress on his or her illness.[28] (See Staudenmayer's chapter in this volume for a more detailed discussion of psychological approaches to treatment.)

TABLE 3. Treatment Recommendations for IEI

Treatment should be individualized but may include the following:
  Nonjudgmental, supportive therapy
  Enhance patient's sense of control
  Reduce psychosocial stress and/or patient's response to stress
  Biofeedback, relaxation response
  Treatment of coexisting psychiatric illness
  Behavioral desensitization to *low-level* chemical exposures
  Pharmacologic treatments to control symptoms
  Increase in physical and social activity
  Specific treatment for hyperventilation (paper bag, respirator)
  Treatment of other coexisting medical illnesses

From Sparks PJ, Daniell W, Black DW, et al: Multiple chemical sensitivity syndrome: A clinical perspective. II. Evaluation, diagnostic testing, treatment, and social considerations. J Occup Med 36(7):731–737, 1994; with permission.

A multidisciplinary and behavioral medicine approach similar to that taken in the treatment of chronic pain, chronic fatigue syndrome, or fibromyalgia, which also may not have objective physical correlates, may help the patient better cope with his or her symptoms.[16] The fundamental principle of behavioral approaches is **symptom desensitization** by gradually increasing exposure in an organized program allowing for accommodation and increasing tolerance.[10]

Any behavioral program also should promote an overall increase in physical and social activity. There are few published reports related to such desensitization treatments for IEI, but clinical experiences suggests that the efficacy of this approach warrants controlled study.[2,10,11,25] This approach assumes that an important contributing factor to the manifestation of IEI is primarily behavioral without associated objective or progressive physiologic impairment, dysfunction, and disease. Provocation chamber challenges under double-blinded placebo-controlled conditions may have therapeutic value in selected patients[30,31] as part of this process.

Researchers in Sweden[3] found in a controlled study of 17 randomly assigned IEI patients (reporting sensitivity to electricity) that cognitive-behavioral therapy was effective in reducing self-reports of functional disability. Double-blind provocation tests also indicated that the IEI patients could not reliably distinguish between the presence or absence of the putative environmental cause of their symptoms.

Enhancing the patient's sense of control over workplace or home stressors, including environmental chemical exposures, is likely to be effective in managing symptoms. A variety of approaches to reducing stress in the IEI patient exist, and many do not involve treatment by a mental health professional or physician. These may include massage, physical therapy, prayer, meditation, or regular exercise, for example.

Systematic changes in the organization of work may be needed to reduce organizational stress. Odors and exposure to volatile organic compounds in the workplace and home that are perceived as irritating or noxious by the symptomatic individual should be reduced and controlled as much as possible. This should be attempted even if levels of exposure are below government-mandated or recommended permissible exposure limits. It is necessary, although challenging, to balance the benefits of the above recommendations with the potential risks of a spiraling pattern of progressively severe environmental restrictions and loss of employment.

Importantly, treatment of coexisting psychiatric manifestations, such as depression and panic attacks, is likely to reduce symptoms and disability.[25,31] Psychiatric treatments may be helpful in controlling symptoms *regardless* of etiology. Even if specific immunologic, neurophysiological, or neurotoxic mechanisms are ultimately discovered to be operative in some patients with IEI, treatment of psychiatric symptoms may still be a most effective approach to palliation.

For those patients in whom hyperventilation and anxiety may be playing a major role in their symptoms, instruction in techniques such as re-breathing into a paper bag are helpful. Some such patients have noted improvement in symptoms with the wearing of a respirator, which increases the dead space and raises blood CO_2.[18,20]

As most patients given a diagnosis of IEI resist the idea that psychological factors play any role at all in their distress, it may be helpful to co-manage such patients with a primary-care physician experienced in the diagnosis and treatment of depression, anxiety, and somatiform disorders, rather than a psychiatrist. The goal of treatment at this time must be relief of symptoms, rather than expectation of cure.[28]

Pharmacologic treatment may be a helpful adjunct in relief of the psychophysiologic symptoms, such as depression and mood swings, chronic fatigue, difficulty sleeping, and anxiety, that accompany chemical sensitivity—regardless of the etiology of those symptoms. Certainly, those who meet DSM-IV criteria for major depression should be considered for a trial of antidepressant medication, but psychopharmacologic drugs should be prescribed only as part of an overall treatment program, ideally involving an expert in mental health. However, many patients with IEI report intolerance to relatively low doses of any medication or "chemical" intervention, and this needs to be considered in initiating antidepressant therapy. Despite these obvious challenges, the rewards from successfully uncovering and relieving depression, anxiety, and mood swings justify the effort.

Those patients who completely deny that stress or psychological factors might play a role in their symptoms, and who perceive the locus of control to be outside themselves, probably cannot be helped by any of the above medical therapies.[30]

Some IEI patients have attempted to pursue bizarre and costly treatments and may appear desperate as they seek unorthodox therapies such as sublingual neutralization, or various "detoxification" treatment programs. While remaining nonjudgmental about the patient's motivation to seek such therapies, it is the physician's responsibility to educate the patient about their lack of efficacy.[1]

A definite medical recommendation for complete avoidance of chemical exposures is not indicated at this time. In fact, since there is no evidence for a cumulative toxic injury underlying IEI, recommendation for long-term avoidance of chemical exposures is contraindicated. It also is impossible to accomplish. One cannot readily remove the IEI patient from chemical exposures if the patient presents with an ever-changing list of exposures of concern which cannot be measured or tested and which result in unpredictable or individually determined responses. Without negating the symptoms, reassure the patient that IEI is not associated with signs of progressive disease, nor is it fatal.

Currently there are no data showing that long-term withdrawal from exposure produces an improvement in symptoms, and there is some data that symptoms become worse.[4,32] Major lifestyle modifications frequently lead to substantial and deleterious consequences, such as loss of work and social support, which may exacerbate or produce depression and anxiety. The burden of proof that avoidance is effective in reducing symptoms and is necessary to prevent toxic injury rests with the proponents.

Finally, IEI has been recognized as a potentially disabling condition by some governmental agencies such as the Social Security Administration and the U.S. Department of Housing and Urban Development. Political or social definitions of IEI as work-related or disabling, however, should not cloud the physician's judgment regarding the diagnosis, attribution, and treatment of symptoms associated with IEI in the individual patient.

REFERENCES

1. American College of Physicians: Position statement: Clinical ecology. Ann Intern Med 111:168–178, 1989.
2. Amundsen MA, Hanson NP, Bruce BK, et al: Odor aversion or multiple chemical sensitivities: A name change and description of successful behavioral medicine treatment. Regul Toxicol Pharmacol 24:S116–S118, 1996.
3. Andersson B, Berg M, Arnetz BB, et al: A cognitive-behavioral treatment of patients suffering from "electric hypersensitivity": Subjective effects and reactions in a double-blind provocation study. J Occup Environ Med 38(8):752–758, 1996.
4. Black D: The relationship of mental disorders and idiopathic environmental intolerance. Occup Med 15(2), 2000.
5. Bolla K: Idiopathic environmental intolerance. Occup Med 15(2), 2000.

6. Council on Scientific Affairs, American Medical Association: Clinical etiology. JAMA 268:3465–3467, 1992.

7. Dalton P: Odor perception and beliefs about risks. Chem Senses 21:447–458, 1996.

8. Daniell WE, Stockbridge HL, Labbe RF, et al: Environmental chemical exposures in disturbances of heme synthesis. Environ Health Perspect 105(Suppl1):37–53, 1997.

9. Engel GL: The clinical application of the biopsychosocial model. Am J Psychiatry 137:535–544, 1980.

10. Giardino ND, Lehrer PM: Behavioral conditioning in idiopathic environmental intolerance. Occup Med 15(2), 2000.

11. Guglielmi RS, Cox DJ, Spyker DA: Behavioral treatment of phobic avoidance in multiple chemical sensitivity. J Behav Ther Exp Psychiatry 25:197–209, 1994.

12. Haller E: Successful management of patients with "multiple chemical sensitivities" on an inpatient psychiatric unit. J Clin Psychiatry 54:196–199, 1993.

13. Hahn M, Bonkovsky HL: Multiple chemical sensitivity syndrome and porphyria. Arch Intern Med 157:281–285, 1997.

14. Hill AB: The environment and disease: Association or causation? Proc R Soc Med 58:295–300, 1965.

15. Hu H, Johnson K: A report to the State of Washington Department of Labor and Industries: A comparison of single photon emission computed tomography in normal controls, in subjects with multiple chemical sensitivity syndrome, and in subjects with chronic fatigue syndrome. 1999.

16. Institute of Medicine: Pain and Disability. Washington, D.C., National Academy Press, 1987.

17. Jewett DL, Fein G, Greenberg MH: A double-blind study of symptom provocation to determine food sensitivity. N Engl J Med 343:429–433, 1990.

18. Leznoff A: Clinical aspects of allergic disease: provocation challenges in patients with multiple chemical sensitivity. J Allery Clin Immunol 99(4):438–442, 1997.

19. Leznoff A: Personal communication. 1997

20. Leznoff A, Binkley KE: Idiopathic environmental intolerance: Results of challenge studies. Occup Med 15(2), 2000.

21. Margolick J: Immune diagnostic tests. Personal communication and presentations at a conference entitled Chemicals, the Environment, and Disease: A Research Perspective. Sponsored by the Washington Department of Labor and Industry, May 7, 1999. Seattle, WA.

22. Reference deleted.

23. Nuwer MR: On the controversies about clinical use of EEG brain mapping. Brain Topogr 3:103–111, 1990.

24. Salvaggio JE: Understanding clinical immunological testing in alleged chemically induced environmental illnesses. Regul Toxicol Pharmacol 24(1):S16–S27, 1996.

25. Simon GE: Psychiatric treatment in MCS. Toxicol Ind Health 8:221–228, 1992.

26. Simon G, Daniell W, Stockbridge H, et al: Immunologic, psychological, and neuropsychological factors in multiple chemical sensitivity: A controlled study. Ann Intern Med 119:97–103, 1993.

27. Society of Nuclear Medicine Brain Imaging Council: The ethical clinical practice of functional brain imaging. J Nucl Med 37(7):1256–1259, 1996.

28. Sparks PJ, Daniell W, Black DW, et al: Multiple chemical sensitivity syndrome: A clinical perspective. II. Evaluation, diagnostic testing, treatment, and social considerations. J Occup Med 36(7):731–737, 1994.

29. Staudenmayer H, Selner JC, Buhr MP: Double-blind provocation chamber challenges in 20 patients presenting with "multiple chemical sensitivity." Regul Toxicol Pharmacol 18:44–53, 1993.

30. Staudenmayer H: Clinical consequences of the EI/MCS "diagnosis:" Two paths. Reg Toxicol Pharmacol 24(1):S96–110, 1996.

31. Staudenmayer H: Psychological treatment of psychogenic idiopathic environmental intolerance. Occup Med 15(2), 2000.

32. Terr AI: Environmental illness: A clinical review of 50 cases. Arch Intern Med 146:145–149, 1986.

33. Terr AI: Immunological issues in "multiple chemical sensitivities." Reg Toxicol Pharmacol 18:54–60, 1993.

34. Waxman AD: Functional brain imaging in the assessment of multiple chemical sensitivities. Occup Med 15(2), 2000.

35. Weaver VM: Medical management of the multiple chemical sensitivity patient. Reg Toxicol Pharmacol 24(1):S111–S115, 1996.

ALAN D. WAXMAN, MD

FUNCTIONAL BRAIN IMAGING IN THE ASSESSMENT OF MULTIPLE CHEMICAL SENSITIVITIES

From Cedars-Sinai Medical Center
Los Angeles, California

Reprint requests to:
Alan D. Waxman, MD
Cedars-Sinai Medical Center
Imaging-Nuclear Medicine
8700 Beverly Blvd.
Room A041
Los Angeles, CA 90048

Imaging of the brain can be accomplished using several techniques. Cross-sectional anatomic imaging usually is done with computed tomography (CT) or magnetic resonance imaging (MRI). Until recently, little or no information about the function of the brain was available, but these cross-sectional imaging tests give exquisite anatomic information. Functional MRI has been used as a research tool in evaluating brain function by measuring increased venous oxygenation following activation. The technique has promise in tumor surgical planning as well as in assessing cerebral vascular reserve in patients following stroke; however, currently it is still a research tool.

Traditionally, functional activity of the brain has been assessed using the nuclear medicine techniques of positron emission tomography (PET) or single photon emission computed tomography (SPECT). Functional brain imaging using PET generally employs the radiopharmaceutical fluorine-18 deoxyglucose (FDG). This pharmaceutical is a glucose analog that is transported across the membrane of the neuron and concentrates mainly in gray matter. The FDG is phosphorelated, but cannot be metabolized through the normal glucose metabolic pathways because of its deoxy formulation. Exceptionally high concentrations of FDG normally are seen in the gray matter of the brain and, to a lesser extent, the white matter. FDG is a positron-emitting isotope that is produced using a cyclotron. Commercial availability is increasing, and FDG may some day be commonly used to produce glucose metabolic maps of the brain.

Recently, there has been a major increase in the number of detectors sold to the medical community which can perform functional brain imaging using coincidence techniques. Due to lack of reimbursement for brain FDG imaging and other factors, most of the functional brain imaging in the United States, Europe, Canada and Japan is done using SPECT techniques.

There are two FDA-approved, commercially available radiopharmaceuticals used for functional brain imaging. These include Tc-99m-hexamethylpropyle-neamine oxime (HMPAO) or Tc-99m-sodium bicisate, also known as ethyl cystinate dimer (ECD). Both of these agents are referred to as brain perfusion agents. They measure perfusion of the brain as well as the ability of the neuronal cell membrane to transport the lipophiloic materials into the neuron, where they then become hydrophiloic and essentially are trapped within the neuron. The distributions of HMPAO and ECD are similar, but not identical. The patterns observed with the use of perfusion agents also are similar, but not identical, to FDG distribution.

The anatomic information offered by the modern-day PET scan approaches the resolution of CT or MRI. The resolution of SPECT is slightly decreased compared to PET; however, comparable diagnostic information is obtained using either PET or SPECT if the studies are done properly with state-of-the-art detectors.

COMPONENTS OF THE PET OR SPECT EXAMINATION

There are six basic components of the PET or SPECT examination. These include: (1) patient preparation, (2) data acquisition, (3) data analysis, (4) data display, (5) interpretation, and (6) reporting.[1]

The most important aspect of patient preparation is to achieve a consistent environment at the time of injection and uptake of the radiopharmaceutical. The acquisition of data is somewhat complex for both PET and SPECT acquisitions. However, with meticulous attention to detail, high-quality images can be produced if the detection equipment is state-of-the-art. Care must be taken to ensure that the patient does not move during the study. Appropriate methods for attenuation correction during the data acquisition phase must be employed. Appropriate algorithms for data processing must be employed for both image production and image analysis, or artifactual results will be produced. Appropriate displays must be utilized to evaluate the data. Highly contrasted color scales are discouraged, since artifactual irregularities may be produced. Interpretation of results should be done by experienced observers who are well versed in the variations that may normally be seen in individuals without disease. In addition, interpretation should be done using accepted techniques of analysis, whether subjective or quantitative.

Suggested methods for reporting functional brain studies have been published and are generally accepted in the medical community.[1,2]

Accepted Applications of Functional Brain Imaging for Clinical Diagnosis

Accepted applications for SPECT imaging of the brain have been published.[3] In general, the consensus is that functional brain imaging may be used for clinical diagnosis in the areas of stroke, dementia (especially the evaluation of Alzheimer's disease) and epilepsy.[1,2,3] The factors determining accepted use for specific applications include issues such as whether published reports are peer-reviewed, especially with respect to both quantity and quality in a specific area.[3] Recognized authorities for specific applications include the Food and Drug Administration, the Society of Nuclear Medicine, and the American Academy of Neurology. Quality factors for acceptance of a procedure include study design and validation.

Study Design

Much of the literature in brain imaging as applied to new or emerging areas such as multiple chemical sensitivity analysis has been hampered by inadequate study design. Most of the published studies have an inadequate control group of normal subjects. In general, these studies fail to have adequate exclusion criteria and lack sufficient numbers of age-matched subjects for either qualitative or quantitative analysis. Technical factors such as inadequate patient preparation, old or inappropriate instrumentation, poor acquisition techniques, and inappropriate data processing and display routines have been responsible for the variable results in the evaluation of multiple chemical sensitivities or toxic exposure. Analytic methods often are flawed because they use statistical assumptions that ensure abnormality in subjects who truly have no abnormalities present.

It is difficult to validate results of functional brain imaging since standard tissue validation methods used in cancer research, i.e., tissue sampling by biopsy, surgery, or autopsy, generally is not done to establish accuracy of diagnosis in assessment of toxic exposure or multiple chemical sensitivities. Validation typically is done using indirect methods, which are always subject to criticism.

RECENT STUDIES OF SPECT IN MCS

Prior studies using functional brain imaging to specifically evaluate multiple chemical sensitivity syndrome (MCS) are limited.[4] Reports of SPECT abnormalities in patients with toxic chemical exposure and resulting "sensitivity" damage to the brain failed to rigorously define their subject population as having MCS.[5–11] Method-related criticisms for these studies have been discussed, and include study design items such as absence of appropriate age-matched controls, lack of blinded reading, lack of quantitation, and unvalidated methodology.[12–14]

A recent assessment of multiple chemical sensitivities using functional brain imaging was performed by Hu and coworkers.[4] This group compared SPECT imaging in normal controls, subjects with MCS, and subjects with chronic fatigue syndrome. The objective of this study was to determine if SPECT imaging is abnormal or has a characteristic pattern in subjects with MCS.

The study design for this project included a population consisting of 27 normal subjects age-matched with 27 subjects diagnosed as having MCS. MCS subjects were deemed eligible if they met the following criteria:

- Diagnosed with MCS by a board-certified occupational/environmental medicine physician after a full clinical evaluation using Cullen's definition of MCS.
- Symptoms of MCS for a minimum of 6 months.
- No history of any other major disease or illness state that has been associated with central nervous system pathology and /or SPECT scanning abnormalities (e.g., head injury entailing loss of consciousness), cancer (because of potential for brain metastasis), seizure disorder, stroke, Alzheimer's disease, alcoholism, or drug abuse.
- Absence of major depressive disorder, unipolar, as set forth in the American Psychiatric Association's Diagnostic and Statistical Manual of Mental Disorders (DSM-IV).
- Absence of any previous SPECT scan (to minimize selection bias).
- Subject age 20–65 years.
- Not taking any medication known to have a significant impact on cerebral blood flow.

Of importance was a group of 19 patients with a clinical diagnosis of chronic fatigue syndrome (CFS). This group served as a disease control group.

Brain SPECT imaging was performed with a dedicated brain SPECT camera using the radiopharmaceutical Tc-99m ethyl cystinate dimer (Neurolite DuPont). All patients were placed supine, at rest, with eyes open in a darkened room. All were injected with 20 mCi of Tc-99m-ECD. Identical acquisition protocols were used for the normal, MCS, and CFS groups.

Following the data acquisition, the studies were analyzed using a visual analysis by a blinded observer who did not know if he was reading the normal, MCS, or CFS group. Quantitative analysis was performed using either the statistical parametric mapping technique or singular value decomposition. Statistical parametric mapping compares regional relative perfusions between groups on a voxel by voxel basis using t-statistics. The difference values were considered significant when the probability values were less than 0.01. In addition, to provide protection against random errors, pixels had to be in a contiguous group extending over more than one transaxial plane.

The results of this study gave tremendous insight into the problems associated with interpretation of brain SPECT even under the most optimal conditions.

The **qualitative results** demonstrated that the sensitivity for detection of MCS was 73% using the normal control group as the basis for comparison. Specificity was only 58%, indicating a false-positive rate of 42%. This is to say that 42% of the normal population would be incorrectly diagnosed as having MCS using the qualitative criteria. When the CFS disease control group was added to the normal group, and the overall sensitivity for detection of MCS was examined, the figure for sensitivity dropped to 31%, while specificity remained unchanged at 61%.

This suggests that even under the most optimal circumstances, using a dedicated brain SPECT system and highly qualified research personnel and physicians, neither the sensitivity nor the specificity was at a level where visual analysis by experts could be used for diagnosing MCS.

The **quantitative results** demonstrated a statistically significant difference between normals in the region of the anterior cingulate gyrus, as well as the region of the brain ventricles (possibly due to ventricular enlargement). These values were obtained using a highly complex statistical parametric mapping analytic technique.

Using singular value decomposition analysis, it was demonstrated that anatomic features that contributed most to the discriminant weights included reduced global perfusion, enlarged lateral ventricles, and reductions in the frontal perfusion in the ventricular and anterior cingulate regions. These findings were similar to those found using statistical parametric mapping analysis.

Among the MCS cases, 74%, 19%, and 7% were classified as MCS subjects, normal controls, and CFS subjects, respectively. Among the CFS subjects, 90%, 0%, and 10% were classified as CFS subjects, normal controls, and MCS subjects, respectively. Among the normal controls, 67%, 26%, and 7% were classified as normal controls, MCS subjects, and CFS subjects, respectively. While some discrimination of subgroups was demonstrated, a diagnostic overlap appears to be present, especially in the ability to discriminate normals from subjects with MCS. In the normal control group, 33% of normal controls were diagnosed as having either MCS (26%) or CFS (7%).

The limitations of this study, acknowledged by the authors, include:
- No diagnostic gold standard or characteristic tissue pathology exists to identify true MCS cases.

- MCS is difficult to prove; therefore, cases may be a heterogeneous set of disorders including fibromyalgia (this was not assessed as part of the study).
- Psychiatric diagnosis were not excluded (similar findings have been reported in depression, anxiety, obsessive-compulsive disorders, and possibly early frontal lobe dementia).
- The study did not screen for caffeine or other drugs, which are known to have an effect on cerebral perfusion and/or metabolism.

SUMMARY AND CONCLUSIONS

To date, peer-reviewed literature is minimal with respect to the use of brain PET or SPECT in MCS. Study designs in general have been poor, with either no or limited age-matched controls, inappropriate quantitative techniques, and/or unblinded reading, which promotes a reader bias.

The Hu study is an excellent study, but still has limitations as outlined. The visual readings under optimal conditions were not suitable for diagnostic purposes, and had a false-positive rate of 42%. From all studies to date, including that of Hu et al., PET and SPECT do not appear to be suitable methodologies to diagnose MCS. As with other brain PET and SPECT studies, including those of toxic exposure or minor head trauma, the results cannot be validated using appropriate gold standards such as tissue pathology. PET and SPECT appear to be excellent tools for research in MCS; when done with proper quantitative techniques, they may indicate a specific trend or pattern that is difficult to evaluate visually. Future studies may evaluate subjects on a serial basis comparing symptomatic with asymptomatic periods. Comparison with other disorders such as fibromyalgia may be of interest. It is clear that additional research with improved study design—possibly with greater resources—is needed to further evaluate the use of these functional imaging tests in evaluating patients with MCS.

REFERENCES

1. Juni JE, AD Waxman, MD Devous Sr., et al: Procedure Guidelines for Brain Perfusion SPECT Using Technetium-99m Radiopharmaceuticals. J Nucl Med 39:923–926, 1998.
2. Waxman AD: Ethical Clinical Practice of Functional Brain Imaging. J of Nucl Med 37:1256–1259, 1996.
3. Report of the Therapeutics and Technology Assessment Subcommittee of the American Academy of Neurology: Assessment of brain SPECT. Neurology 46:278–285, 1996.
4. Hu H, K Johnson, R Heldman, et al: A Comparison of Single Photon Emission Computed Tomography in Normal Controls, in Subjects with Multiple Chemical Sensitivity Syndrome, and in Subjects with Chronic Fatigue Syndrome. A report to the State of Washington, Dept of Labor and Industries.
5. Heuser G, I Mena, J Goldstein, et al: NeuroSPECT Findings in Patients Exposed to Neurotoxic Chemicals. Clin Nucl Med 18:923, 1993.
6. Callender TJ, L Morrow, K Subramanian, et al: Three- dimensional brain metabolic imaging in patients with toxic encephalopathy. Environ Res 60:295–319, 1993.
7. Heuser G, I Mena, F Alamos: NeuroSPECT Findings in Patients Exposed to Neurotoxic Chemicals. Tox Ind Health 10:561–571, 1994.
8. Simon TR, DC Hickey, CE Fincher, et al: Single Photon Emission Tomography of the Brain in Patients with Chemical Sensitivity Syndrome. Scand J Rheumatol 26:364–367, 1997.
9. Fincher CE, TS Chang, EH Harrell, et al: Comparison of Single Photon Emission Computed Tomography Findings in Cases of Healthy Adults and Solvent-exposed Adults. Am J Ind Med 31:813–827, 1998.
10. Heuser G, I Mena: NeuroSPECT in Neurotoxic Chemical Exposure: Demonstration of Long-term Functional Abnormalities. Tox Ind Health 14:813–827, 1998.
11. Ross GH, WJ Rea, AR Johnson, et al: Environmental Health Center. Toxicol Ind Health 15:415–420, 1999.

12. Mayberg H: Response panel #4. Proceedings of the Conference on Low-level Exposure to Chemicals and Neurobiologic Sensitivity. Toxicol Ind Health 10:597–603, 1994.
13. Franzblau A, S Minoshima, TG Robins, DH Garabrant: Comparison of Single Photon Emission Computed Tomography Findings in Cases of Healthy Adults and Solvent-Exposed Adults (Letter to the Editor). Am J Ind Med 32:695–697, 1997.
14. Mayberg HS: Functional Brain Scans as Evidence in Criminal Court: An Argument for Caution. J Nucl Med 33(6):18N–25N, 1992.

KAREN I. BOLLA, PhD

USE OF NEUROPSYCHOLOGICAL TESTING IN IDIOPATHIC ENVIRONMENTAL INTOLERANCE

From Johns Hopkins University
Department of Neurology
Baltimore, Maryland

Reprint requests to:
Karen I. Bolla, PhD
Johns Hopkins Bayview Medical
    Center
Department of Neurology
A Building, Room 672
Baltimore, MD 21224

This chapter is intended to provide the reader with information so that he/she can decide the usefulness of a neuropsychological evaluation in the assessment of individuals with idiopathic environmental intolerance (IEI). It is important to understand the types of questions the neuropsychological assessment can answer and, perhaps even more important, cannot answer.

NEUROPSYCHOLOGICAL ASSESSMENT

Historically, a neuropsychological assessment consisted of examiner-administered oral and written tests. More recently, computerized tests have been introduced into the test battery. Advantages of computerized testing include standardization in administration, greater measurement precision for timed tasks (i.e., reaction time), reductions in scoring errors, and ease of data collection in large epidemiologic studies. Disadvantages of computerized testing include limited human interaction, which can result in reduced motivation leading to suboptimal performance; an inability to assess verbal skills without sophisticated computer software; and a paucity of normative values for various populations.

A well-constructed neuropsychological test battery assesses the spectrum of cognitive domains, including intelligence, orientation, attention/concentration, language, remote memory, verbal and visual short-term memory, visuoconstruction/perception, executive/psychomotor functioning, manual dexterity, and affect. Also, convergent validity is measured by giving multiple

TABLE 1. Examples of Neuropsychological Tests

Intellectual Ability	**Psychological Functioning—Mood**
Wechsler Adult Intelligence Scale, 3rd ed. (WAIS-III)	Minnesota Multiphasic Personality Inventory-2 (MMPI-2)
Vocabulary—WAIS-III	Symptom Checklist (SCL-90-R)
Shipley Institute of Living Scale	Profile of Mood States (POMS)
Raven's Progressive Matrices	Center for Epidemiologic Studies Depression
Language	Scale (CES-D)
Boston Naming Test	**Memory**
Peabody Picture Vocabulary Test-Revised (PPVT-R)	Wechsler Memory Scale, 3rd ed. (WMS-III)
	Verbal Memory
Wide Range Achievement Test (WRAT-3)	Rey Auditory Verbal Learning Test (RAVLT)
Reading and Spelling Subtests	California Verbal Learning Test (CVLT)
Boston Diagnostic Aphasia Examination (BDAE)	Logical Memory Passages—WMS-III
	Nonverbal Memory
Western Aphasia Battery (WAB)	Visual Reproduction—WMS-III
Manual Dexterity/Motor	Rey-Osterrieth Complex Figure Test
Purdue Pegboard	Symbol Digit Paired Associate Learning Test
Grooved Pegboard	**Visuoconstruction/Visuoperception**
Finger Tapping Test	Rey-Osterrieth Complex Figure Test
Executive/Psychomotor Functions	Judgement of Line Orientation
Wisconsin Card Sorting Test	Hooper Visual Organization Test
Category Test	Block Design—WAIS-III
Stroop	**Computerized Batteries**
Digit Symbol—WAIS-III	Neurobehavioral Evaluation System (NES-2)
Symbol Digit Modalities Test	Milan Automated Neuropsychological System
Trail Making Test	(MANS - WHO)
Reaction Time	Automated Neuropsychological Assessment
Continuous Performance Test	Metrics (ANAM)

tests that evaluate the same cognitive domain. For example, when abnormal test results are observed on only one of three verbal memory tests, then a memory deficit is less likely since a conclusion of a neurologic deficit in a specific cognitive domain requires substantial agreement among the results of two or more measures. Numerous standardized tests are available that measure level of performance in each cognitive domain (Table 1). These tests are described in two excellent sources.[10,13]

Since symptoms of affective disorders can mimic the symptoms of CNS dysfunction, it is important to rule out anxiety and/or depressive disorders before diagnosing a neurologic deficit. Such exclusion can be accomplished through the use of the clinical interview and a variety of standardized questionnaires, such as the Center for Epidemiological Studies - Depression Scale (CES-D),[14] the Symptom Checklist-90-Revised (SCL-90-R),[6] and the Minnesota Multiphasic Personality Inventory (MMPI and MMPI - 2).[9]

INTERPRETATION OF TEST RESULTS— LIMITATIONS/CAUTIONS

Absence of a Biomarker

Accurate determination of exposure to a neurotoxicant requires availability of a biomarker. Unfortunately, with the exception of the heavy metals, there are few readily available biomarkers. Without a biomarker, it is difficult to determine if the magnitude or intensity of exposure was sufficient to cause alterations in the central nervous system (CNS; dose-response relationship). The evaluation of patients with IEI is especially problematic because there are no biomarkers and therefore no established dose-response relationships. In addition, it is unclear if exposures to environmental irritants even produce adverse neurobehavioral effects. Therefore, it is impossible to determine with a high degree of certainty if neurobehavioral findings are related to chemical exposure in patients who present with symptoms of IEI.

Neuropsychological assessment, although limited in its specificity, is the best method for detecting adverse effects of neurotoxicants on the CNS. Lead, organic solvents, mercury, manganese, carbon disulfide, carbon monoxide, herbicides, and pesticides are all known neurotoxicants. In contrast, many other chemicals reported to cause symptoms in patients presenting with IEI generally are not classified as neurotoxicants, but rather as irritants. Epidemiologic studies on the neurobehavioral effects of neurotoxicants provide scientific data on which to base our clinical interpretations. However, there is no rigorous scientific data on the neurobehavioral effects of irritants, only anecdotal reports. This makes the clinical interpretation of findings in patients with IEI difficult.

Adequate Normative Values for Reference

Speculation about the cause of poor performance on a neurobehavioral test must be made with caution. To determine if a score falls outside the normal range, adequate norms must be used for comparison. For example, intellectual ability predicts test performance to a large extent, but few norms are currently available for individuals with low levels or high levels of intellectual functioning. Comparing the test results of an individual with low intellectual ability with normative values based on a more intelligent group would lead to the erroneous conclusion of CNS injury where none exists. Conversely, performance decrements in highly intelligent people may be missed, since even their diminished performance may still meet or exceed the upper limits of a normative group representing a more average level of intellectual functioning. In addition, cognitive performance also is influenced by age and sex.[2] Therefore, to ensure an accurate diagnosis, the clinician must use norms that have been modified to include the effects of modifying variables such as intelligence, age, and sex (Table 2).

Interpretation of Test Results—Differential Diagnoses

The validity of test results must be determined when abnormal neurobehavioral performance is found. For example, if a deficit is truly a result of an alteration in brain functioning, outcomes of more than one test of the same cognitive domain (e.g., verbal memory) should be abnormal. Also, performance on more difficult tasks should not be better than on easier tests, and performance within tests should decline as the test progresses from easier to more difficult items. Specific patterns of performance across all the tests provide information on the nature of brain injury (e.g., static versus progressive, acute versus chronic, diffuse versus localized). Significant performance deterioration after removal from the source of chemical exposure is uncharacteristic of brain injury due to neurotoxicants. Instead, a progressive disease process like Alzheimer's disease should be ruled out. When test results show a decline in a specific cognitive domain that is inconsistent with the individual's general level of intelligence as determined by other test results, school records, or occupational history, then an acute process is likely and would be consistent with a neurotoxic insult. However, this pattern also may be consistent with a host of other neurologic disorders (Table 3). Specific patterns of performance also can be used to determine if brain injury is diffuse or localized. If findings can be localized (e.g., only

TABLE 2.   Age, Sex, and Vocabulary Score: Effects on Neuropsychological Test Performance

Test	Age	Sex	Vocabulary Score
Vocabulary	**		
Similarities			***
Controlled Verbal Fluency (FAS)		*	***
Verbal - Verbal IV	***	*	
Rey Auditory Verbal Learning, Trial V	***	***	
RAVLT Recognition		*	
RAVLT Intrusions		***	
Logical Memory Immediate			***
Logical Memory Delayed	***	***	***
Serial Digit Learning	***		
Symbol Digit Paired Associate Learning	***	*	**
Visual Reproduction	***		
Block Design	***	*	*
Trails A	***		
Trails B	***		
Digit Symbol	***	*	*
Consonant Trigrams	**	*	***
Reaction Time, Truncated Mean	***	***	
Reaction Time, Minimum	***	***	
Purdue, Dominant	***	***	
Purdue, Nondominant	***	*	
Purdue, Both Hands	***		
Purdue, Assembly	***	*	

(*) $p < 0.05$; (**) $p < 0.01$, (***) $p < 0.001$

TABLE 3.   Disorders Associated with Neuropsychological Findings

Neurologic Disorders	**Medical Disorders**
Alzheimer's disease	Cardiopulmonary illness
Anoxic brain injury	Diabetes
Acquired immunodeficiency syndrome—	Hepatic disease
AIDS dementia	Renal disease
Cerebrovascular disease	Sjorgren's disease
Development disability	Sleep disorders
Attentional deficit disorder	Systemic lupus erythematosus
Learning disability	Thyroid dysfunction
Epilepsy	**Neuropsychiatric Disorders**
Head injury	Anxiety disorders
Huntington's disease	Obsessive-compulsive disorder
Multi-infarct dementia	Panic attacks
Multiple sclerosis	Post-traumatic stress disorder
Normal pressure hydrocephalus	Somatoform disorder
Parkinson's disease	Depression
Pernicious anemia	
Progressive supranuclear palsy	
Toxic encephalopathies	
Heavy metals	
Chemical toxins	
Medications	
Alcohol, drugs of abuse	
Viral and nonviral CNS infections	
Withdrawal syndromes	

language deficits), then toxic encephalopathy is unlikely, and an EEG and/or MRI is indicated. Adverse effects of chemicals on the CNS are static, acute, and diffuse.

Neurobehavioral tests have **high sensitivity**, but **low specificity**. It is important to determine if cognitive decrements are related to chemical exposure or to another CNS, medical, or neuropsychiatric disorder. Although patients may report a recent onset of cognitive difficulties, review of school records and prior employment evaluations might indicate longstanding problems (i.e., subnormal intelligence or learning disability). Depression or anxiety also can produce decrements in neuropsychological test performance. These decrements usually are observed in the areas of attention, learning and memory, and psychomotor speed. Since similar cognitive domains are affected by both neurotoxicants and alterations in mood, it often is difficult to determine the relative contribution of each to decrements in neuropsychological test performance. More specifically, such symptomatology could be related to neurotoxic exposure, the emotional state and personality characteristics of the patient, or to some combination of the three. In order to determine the etiology of complaints, patterns of performance and inconsistencies during testing (such as superior performance on harder tasks, with poor performance on easier ones, or lower than chance performance on all of the tasks) must be examined carefully.

Neurotoxicants have not been associated with decrements in any aspect of language (reading, writing, naming, speech), or in remote memory. Remote memory is assessed by asking questions concerning significant early life experiences. With the exception of acute, high-level exposure, disorientation is not characteristic of neurotoxicant exposure. Therefore, if any of the above symptoms are reported, it is unlikely that chemical exposure is responsible for these symptoms.

Repetitive testing may be helpful when making the differential diagnosis. If psychological mechanisms are suspected, repeat testing over a short time interval (days) will provide information on the stability of the findings. If there are large discrepancies between the results of the two batteries, alterations in affective state are most likely responsible. If performance decrements are physiological, then performance should remain constant or improve if there has been little or no chemical exposure during the test-retest interval. If performance deteriorates significantly without re-exposure, then a progressive disease or secondary psychological reaction to the exposure should be suspected.

NEUROPSYCHOLOGICAL DECREMENTS IN INDIVIDUALS WITH IEI

It has been postulated that a wide variety of chemicals cause neurophysiologic alterations in patients with IEI. If this is true, then the same constellation of cognitive deficits should be present or absent in persons with IEI as in persons with documented neurotoxic exposure. Epidemiologic studies have reported decrements in attention/concentration, new learning and memory, executive/psychomotor speed, and manual dexterity in individuals exposed to organic solvents.[1,3] However, few if any neurobehavioral decrements have been reported in individuals with IEI. Fiedler et al.[7] found performance abnormalities on one test of verbal memory in a group of IEI patients who had been carefully selected for not having a history of psychiatric disorder. No other performance abnormalities were indicated. Similarly, Simon et al.[12] reported no differences in neuropsychological test performance between individuals with IEI and controls (patients with musculoskeletal injuries). In another study in subjects with sensitivities to chemicals, performance on standardized neuropsychological tests did not substantiate the subjects' subjective reports of cognitive impairment.[8]

Neurobehavioral functioning was evaluated in 35 chemically exposed patients referred to an Occupational and Environmental Neurology Clinic.[3] Of these 35 patients, 17 presented with symptoms of IEI, and 16 patients reported no symptoms of IEI. In addition, a group of 126 healthy controls was used for comparison. The performance of the IEI group was not significantly different from the control group on tests of verbal learning and memory, executive functioning, and psychomotor functioning. In fact, chemically exposed patients with symptoms of IEI outperformed a group of patients with similar chemical exposures but without symptoms of IEI. While the IEI group performed below the control group on a test of visual learning and memory, this performance was similar to the group with chemical exposure without IEI. Therefore, performance on objective neurobehavioral tests did not confirm the most frequently reported subjective complaints of patients with IEI. These findings suggest no permanent impairment of brain function in IEI patients. Alternative explanations could be that the neurobehavioral tests used in the examination were not sensitive enough to detect the types of cognitive difficulties experienced by IEI patients, or that cognitive deficits only became apparent during exposure to chemicals. These explanations are unlikely since many of the patients reported chronic, severe limitations in their activities of daily living (ADLs). Neurocognitive deficits that are severe enough to cause changes in ADLs should be detectable on neuropsychological testing.

POSSIBLE AFFECTIVE DISTURBANCES IN INDIVIDUALS WITH IEI

Neuropsychiatric disturbance may be a primary or secondary sequella of chemical exposure. Emotional reactions to exposure may be as important or more important than the direct physiological effects of the chemicals, especially when considering etiology and persistence of symptoms. The fear associated with suspected exposures can be stressful enough to cause severe mental disorders such as somatoform disorders, anxiety disorders, adjustment disorders, and typical and atypical post-traumatic stress disorders. In addition, specific inherent personality characteristics may predispose an individual to develop physical, cognitive, and psychological symptoms.

Using the Minnesota Multiphasic Personality Inventory (MMPI), individuals who present with IEI tend to show a pattern consistent with obsessive-compulsive personality styles. This clinical finding suggests that perfectionistic, obsessive-compulsive personality types may be hypersensitive to endogenous stimuli. Expectations by susceptible individuals that exposure to chemicals has adversely affected their health may result in enhanced awareness of normal bodily sensations. This normal physiological activity may then be misinterpreted as abnormal physical, cognitive, and affective symptoms. The cause of these symptoms is then misattributed to chemical exposure (Figs. 1 and 2). This theoretical model applies to exposure to toxic as well as non-toxic chemicals.

With acute, high-level chemical exposure, physical symptoms appear to be immediate, prominent, and primary. Other primary symptoms may include alterations in mood and cognitive symptoms such as acute confusional states. In contrast, with chronic, low-level chemical exposure, the most prominent symptoms appear to be alterations in mood and cognition. The interaction between mood and cognition appears to be stronger than with acute chemical exposures. The degree an individual is hypersensitive to endogenous stimuli (normal bodily sensations) may determine the duration and intensity of symptoms.

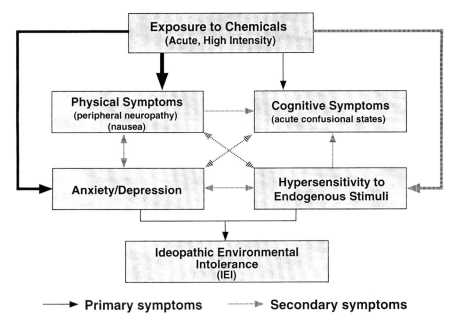

FIGURE 1. The development and persistence of physical, cognitive, and affective symptoms following *acute, high-intensity,* chemical exposure in individuals with IEI. Solid lines = primary symptoms; dotted lines = secondary symptoms.

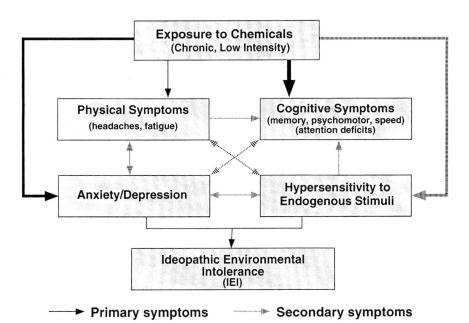

FIGURE 2. The development and persistence of physical, cognitive, and affective symptoms following *chronic, low-intensity,* chemical exposure in individuals with IEI. Solid lines = primary symptoms; dotted lines = secondary symptoms.

Furthermore, in a subgroup of exposed individuals, distressing symptoms may continue to be experienced because these symptoms have been conditioned.[5,12] This conditioning adheres to a Pavlovian conditioning model in which symptoms are an unconditioned or naturally occurring response to exposure to an odorous chemical. The association of the odor of the toxicant with the symptoms of the exposure causes classical conditioning of the strong odor alone, which can serve in the future as a conditioned stimulus (CS), eliciting the same symptoms as the chemical itself. Repeated or prolonged exposure strengthens the conditioned association between odor and illness. When generalization of a response occurs, a different odor (CS) will elicit the same response as the original stimulus.

SUMMARY
The neuropsychological evaluation provides unique information on the functional integrity of the CNS. As with any diagnostic process, the ability to pinpoint the diagnosis among neurotoxicant exposure, neurologic disease, medical illness, or neuropsychiatric disturbance is based on the combined evidence taken from the medical, occupational, social, and academic histories, physical and neurologic exams, biological monitoring, EEG, CT/MRI, and the neuropsychological evaluation.

When evaluating patients who present with symptoms of IEI, it is irresponsible to routinely attribute their symptoms to the presence of a neuropsychiatric disorder. It is equally irresponsible to attribute IEI-like symptoms to chemical exposure without rigorously exploring other etiologies. If other causes for the symptoms are not considered, then many treatable conditions will remain unidentified and untreated. Finally, the neuropsychological evaluation cannot be used to diagnose IEI, but rather should be used to rule out treatable causes for the symptoms experienced by the patient with IEI.

ACKNOWLEDGMENTS

The author thanks Eugene R. Valendo, M.S., Regina Galante, B.A., and Maria Mouratidis, M.A. for their thoughtful comments and editorial input.

REFERENCES
1. Bleecker ML, Bolla KI, Agnew J, et al: Dose-related neurobehavioral effects of chronic exposure to low levels of organic solvents. Am J Ind Med 19:715–728, 1991.
2. Bolla K: Neuropsychological assessment for detecting adverse effects of volatile organic compounds on the central nervous system. Environ Health Perspect 95:93–98, 1991.
3. Bolla KI: Neurobehavioral performance in Multiple Chemical Sensitivities. Regul Toxicol Pharmacol 24:S52–S54, 1995.
4. Bolla KI, Schwartz BS, Stewart W, et al: Comparison of neurobehavioral function in workers exposed to a mixture of organic and inorganic lead and in workers exposed to solvents. Am J Ind Med 27:231–246, 1995.
5. Bolla-Wilson K, Wilson RJ, Bleecker ML: Conditioning of physical symptoms after neurotoxic exposure. J Occup Med 30:684–686, 1988.
6. Derogatis LR: SCL-90 administration, scoring, and procedures manual. Baltimore, Johns Hopkins, 1977.
7. Fieldler N, Maccia C, Kipen H: Evaluation of chemically sensitive patients. J Occup Med 34:529–538, 1992.
8. Fiedler N, Kipen HM, DeLuca J, et al: A controlled comparison of multiple chemical sensitivities and chronic fatigue syndrome. Psychosom Med 58:38–49, 1996.
9. Green RL: The MMPI-2/MMPI: An Interpretive Manual. Needham Heights, Massachusetts, Allyn and Bacon, 1991.
10. Lezak MD: Neuropsychological Assessment. New York, Oxford University Press, 1995.
11. Shusterman D, Balmes J, Cone J: Behavioral sensitization to irritants/odorants after acute overexposure. J Occup Med 30:565–567, 1988.

12. Simon G, Daniell W, Stockbridge H, et al: Immunologic, psychological, and neuropsychological factors in Multiple Chemical Sensitivity. Ann Intern Med 119:97–103, 1993.
13. Spreen O, Strauss E: A Compendium of Neuropsychological Tests. New York, Oxford University Press, 1991.
14. Weissman MM, Sholomskas D, Pottenger M, et al: Assessing depressive symptoms in five psychiatric populations: A validation study. Am J Epidemiol 106:203–214, 1977.

HERMAN STAUDENMAYER, Ph.D.

PSYCHOLOGICAL TREATMENT OF PSYCHOGENIC IDIOPATHIC ENVIRONMENTAL INTOLERANCE

From Behavioral Medicine and
 Biofeedback Clinic of
 Denver, PC.
Denver, Colorado

Reprint requests to:
Herman Staudenmayer, Ph.D.
Behavioral Medicine and
 Biofeedback Clinic of
 Denver, P.C.
5800 East Evans Avenue
Denver, CO 80222

Prior to considering psychological treatment, several questions need to be answered for each patient presenting with multisystem symptoms attributed to environmental exposures, what is now called idiopathic environmental intolerance (IEI):

- Is IEI essentially a psychogenic psychosocial phenomenon?
- Who advocates unsubstantiated theories and practices?
- Why was the patient at risk to acquire IEI?
- What psychosocial factors perpetuate symptoms and disability?
- How can the physician broach psychogenic issues?

IS IEI PSYCHOGENIC?

This question is addressed elsewhere in this volume (see chapters by Black and by Binkley and Leznoff), and in another book by this author.[95] The recognition of diseases resulting from exposure to toxic levels of chemicals and other environmental agents is undisputed. The pain, suffering, and disability caused by toxicogenic disorders can leave the patient mired in the depths of depression, feeling helpless and grieving lost functioning, or immobilized by anxiety of an uncertain future for self and loved ones. Accordingly, supportive psychotherapy for such patients is well characterized and appropriate. Since IEI is not a validated toxicogenic disease resulting in impairment,[68] but presents as an amorphous constellation of medically unexplained symptoms without objective signs or biological markers, no attempt is made here to describe a strategy for supportive psychotherapy for well-established diseases.

Rather, the focus here is on psychotherapy for patients who suffer from IEI that they believe mimics toxicogenic or other diseases, but is psychogenic like other functional somatic syndromes.[10] Numerous clinical case series[2,17,18,24,47,59,72,82-86,93,101,102,110] and case-control studies[19,20,63,70,92,97-99] corroborate a psychogenic theory of IEI. IEI patients are psychologically heterogeneous, with each individual case defined by a milieu of psychological, psychophysiological, and social factors. Despite this heterogeneity, some common characteristics have been gleaned from this author's clinical experience with several hundred IEI patients (Table 1). While IEI patients believe their symptoms and disability are caused and exacerbated by low-level environmental exposures tolerated by the rest of the population, there are alternative explanations for their symptoms and attributions.

Feelings of helplessness, hopelessness, and loss-of-control accompanied by overt signs and symptoms of depression may reflect despair over low self-esteem. Anxiety and phobias about environmental exposures often symbolize displaced personal anxieties unrelated to environmental intolerances. Physiologic state reactions

TABLE 1. Some IEI Patient Characteristics Exemplified by Patient Statements

EMOTIONS

• Depression, loss of self-image and low self-esteem.
  "IEI takes away the motivation to fight the pain."
  "There is no one to blame. Why was I born."

• Feelings of helplessness, hopelessness, and loss of control.
  "There is nothing I can do about it; I can't be fixed."
  "Fighting back would be futile because people don't understand."

• Anxiety and phobias about being environmentally exposed.
  "I feel panicky in situations and places that don't bother other people."
  "I can't relax; I'm vigilant all the time."

• Displaced anger and rage.   "I am angry at the world for not seeing my suffering."

• Self-pity, victimization, and grieving the loss of happiness.
  "I have so much I want out of life which I could have, were it not for IEI."
  "I don't have a choice about being different, because my body is not working properly."

ISOLATION
• Feelings of being an alien in a strange land.   "The doctors don't believe me because my tests are normal, but my body is different."
• Limiting contact to like-minded victims.   "My family and friends avoid me because I have nothing to talk about except my illness."

DISTRESS AND SUFFERING
• Misconceived mind-body dualism about psychophysiological stress responses and psychiatric disorders.   "They think it's all in my head, when it's my body that won't work."

LIMITATIONS/DISABILITY

• Identifying with the victim/invalid.
  "I resent being dependent on others, but my illness leaves me no choice."
  "I cannot fend for myself; therefore, I cannot be expected to accommodate the needs of others."

characteristic of panic attacks explain the reactions mistakenly attributed to environmental triggers[59] and the associated symptoms of shortness of breath, rapid breathing, rapid heart rate, dizziness, lightheaded, chest pain, headaches, dry mouth, muscle weakness, cold and clammy hands, mental confusion, and anxiety.[17]

Anger and rage originating from experiences and perceptions of injustice and betrayal at the hands of significant individuals in their lives may be displaced onto strangers who do not reinforce or accommodate the patient's environmental beliefs. Such behavior illustrates a psychological defense by which the IEI patient is afraid to be assertive with the threatening individuals. The patient usually lacks insight about such fears and instead feels justified in insisting that IEI be accommodated. Perceived perpetual disability serves to justify attitudes and emotions of victimization.

Like patients with other manifestations of somatization,[78,100] where the specific beliefs of attribution are largely determined by particular medical specialists,[71,108] IEI patients worry about how their illness will affect their future, avoid physical exertion, and unnecessarily give up normal daily activities. Some IEI patients withdraw socially, or in the extreme, may isolate themselves in an environment perceived to be less toxic and safe, such as a perceived "safe home" or a porcelaneous steel trailer parked in the wilderness. This self-imposed austerity and associated eccentric behavior may exacerbate feelings of being an alien in a strange and hostile environment. Access to more realistic conceptualizations of distress and suffering are restricted when social contacts are limited to other victims, or when knowledge about their illness is filtered through advocacy groups and environmental physicians with a selective bias to promote the illness.

Lack of insight for the psychological factors that lead to general malaise symptoms contributes to inappropriate self-identification with the victim/invalid who is impaired, requires assistance, and feels entitled to disability benefits. An unrealistic attitude of mind-body dualism reflects misunderstandings about the physiological pathways of stress-responses associated with somatic and psychological symptoms.[29,30,75] IEI patients often think that the suggestion of their benefiting from psychological or psychiatric intervention is ludicrous. Such denial typically is associated with attitudes of absolution from responsibility for self and the needs of family and friends. In the extreme, IEI becomes an obsessive thought process accompanied by compulsive adherence to unsubstantiated treatment rituals that is self consuming. This includes vitamin and mineral supplements, herbal therapy, "organic foods," water from selected springs, sodium and potassium bicarbonate salts and oxygen to ward off reactions, and sauna depuration to remove toxins from the body.

Somatization Phenomena Presenting as IEI

Somatization is defined as a process by which patients inappropriately focus on physical symptoms while psychosocial problems are denied.[14] Somatization often is diagnosed as a somatoform disorder for lack of evidence of disease pathology or physiologic dysfunction underlying symptoms. Somatizing patients no doubt experience distress, although the mechanisms underlying symptoms are associated with psychiatric conditions or are a manifestation of the stress-response and cognitive styles.[8,57] Symptoms of general malaise usually are exaggerated, and may represent amplifications of normal bodily sensations, fatigue, or lapses in cognitive functioning.[12,65] For example, controlled neuropsychological testing studies with IEI patients[21,36,92] have failed to corroborate patients' claims of debilitating effects—labeled "brain fog"—on attention, memory, and other cognitive processes. Somatization also is associated with depression[55,56] and somatoform disorders.[18,24,77]

The **history of somatization** dates to early descriptions of hysteria, at least 4000 years ago.[37,100] Modern historical accounts identify melancholy in the 17th century,[26] neurasthenia in the 19th century,[90] and autointoxication at the turn of the 20th century.[45] Beginning with Theron Randolph's treatment of his wife for depression, fatigue, and fainting in the 1940s, environmental illness (the original name for IEI) became enmeshed in a variety of phenomena associated with somatization.[91] IEI patients have presented with past or current diagnoses including, but not limited to, hypoglycemia, hypothyroidism, food allergies, candidiasis ("yeast connection"), porphyrin abnormalities, electromagnetic sensitivity, chronic fatigue syndrome or myalgic encephalomyelitis, fibromyalgia, pelvic pain, irritable bowel syndrome, and chronic toxic encephalopathy. Advocates interpret all of these not as independent phenomena, but as manifestations of IEI.

Toxicogenic theories of IEI focus on different mechanistic hypotheses associated with certain medical specialties. Historically, environmental illness was associated with allergy and immunology, chronic fatigue syndrome with virology, limbic kindling and toxic encephalopathy with neurology, fibromyalgia with rheumatology, porphyrin abnormalities with hematology, hypoglycemia with endocrinology, and sensitization with psychology. World events provided opportunities to label the same phenomena— without evidence of toxicologic causation—with new names, such as sick building syndrome[5,62] or Gulf War syndrome.[58]

An obvious **taxonomic question** is whether these diverse manifestations of medically unexplained symptoms represent different manifestations of one latent construct or many functional somatic syndromes with unique etiologic factors. Deary[33] conducted psychometric studies on the correlational structure of the lifetime occurrences of self-reported medically unexplained symptoms in five syndrome groups: fibromyalgia, chronic fatigue syndrome, irritable bowel syndrome, somatic depression, and somatic anxiety. Principal-component analysis and latent trait modeling showed that much of what looks to be attributable to specific syndromes is not so. Rather, these syndromes had a common source of variance, a general, higher order, latent factor for medically unexplained symptoms. Deary concluded that a sizable portion of individual differences in occurrences of the five functional somatic syndromes may be sought in a more general source, common to all of them.

Diagnoses of fashionable illnesses based on hypotheses alluding to well-characterized diseases serve to perpetuate the illusion that there is an association with a physiological mechanism (e.g., porphyria or immunology)[104] or an olfactory model of a biologic mechanism (e.g., limbic kindling or time-dependent sensitization).[73] There is no credible scientific evidence to support such an association,[3] and there is not any testable unifying theory for rationally linking IEI to the postulated mechanisms.[50,73,95] IEI, like other fashionable illnesses, is characterized by:

- vague, subjective multisystem complaints
- a lack of objective laboratory findings
- quasi-scientific explanations
- overlap from one fashionable diagnosis to another
- symptoms consistent with depression or anxiety
- denial of psychosocial distress, or attribution of it to the illness.[37]

What is striking about these seemingly diverse phenomena are the commonalities (Table 2). To avoid the scientific refutation of prior toxicogenic formulations and their exclusion by the courts as "junk science," advocates attempt to create credibility by diagnosing recognized ICD-10 disorders (e.g., toxic encephalopathy, fibromyalgia) and

TABLE 2. Commonalities Among Phenomena Attributed to IEI

HISTORY

In studies, predominantly white middle-aged intelligent females
Multisystem, nonspecific symptomatology
Cognitive dysfunction
Lack of objective medical test results supporting the alleged diagnosis
Lack of objective biomarkers
Normal physical examination
Presupposed diagnosis based on advocacy postulates and mechanistic hypotheses
Comorbidity
Symptom focus determined by advocacy physician or group
Significant subjective impairment (work, play, social, interpersonal, and daily activities)

COGNITIVE STYLE

Symptom amplification
Preoccupation with illness
Vigilance toward body sensations and provoking triggers
Overvalued idea about attribution

PSYCHIATRIC CONDITIONS

Comorbid psychiatric illness, attributed to IEI
Premorbid psychiatric disorders, often without history of diagnosis or treatment
Strength of belief in a physical disease (somatization), predicting poor outcome
Nonadherence to medical treatment
Coping by avoidance, withdrawal, or lack of activity

claiming a causal relation to environmental exposures. Such dissembling confuses patients and the public, and undermines the credibility of psychiatric diagnoses and treatment.

WHO ADVOCATES UNFOUNDED THEORIES AND PRACTICES?

Aside from patient resistance, there are iatrogenic obstacles impeding appropriate medical and psychological intervention.[18,24,25,82,94,95] Environmental physicians are quick to diagnose a host of trendy disorders attributed to environmental intolerances without supportive objective evidence. Some may be well intended, but naive; others are malevolent. They provide misinformation from unsubstantiated tests to exploit the patient's search for an "answer" for his or her pain and suffering which does not implicate the self. The attractiveness of the patient's projective defense is proportional to the amount of anxiety the patient is displacing. Those with the deepest anxiety about self-exploration are at greatest risk of embracing mistaken beliefs about environmental sensitivities which allow projection of the cause of their anxiety into the physical world, away from the self.

The psychodynamics of searching for and finding an "understanding environmental doctor" makes the patient vulnerable to medical cults.[35] Under the influence of an environmental physician and the associated patient support groups and advocacy organizations, social mechanisms seen in epidemic hysteria or mass psychogenic illness flourish.[22,31,44] A social mechanism called *convergence* integrates the diverse symptoms experienced by different individuals, as well as the multitude of attributed environmental agents. Through a second social mechanism called *epidemic contagion*, the different subsets of multisystem symptoms experienced by individuals spread to other members of the community, such that all suffer from anything. Status within the medical cult often is determined by the severity of expressed suffering. The empathy associated with membership is forthcoming as long as the patient espouses the toxicogenic dogma and practices the avoidance, depuration, and other rituals. Introduction of new ideas that are nonconfirming of the belief system is reflexively suspect and the messenger demonized as heretical. The patient motivated by deep- seated anxieties that are inhibited from consciousness may displace them by becoming a crusader for the cause, proselytizing others, and echoing and elaborating unfounded theories of "environmental sensitivities" to anyone who will listen, especially members of the scientific community and activist politicians. Through a variety of circumstances, doctors find themselves confronted by an IEI patient who professes to suffer from a debilitating disease of epidemic proportion. Yet a physician who researches the subject runs into diversions, half-truths, advocation—everything but objective data that supports the toxicogenic postulates.

Another obstacle, reinforced by environmental physicians and other advocates, is the suggestion that taking psychotropic medications and seeing a psychiatrist or psychologist is not warranted because the illness is physical, not mental. Adherence to psychiatric or psychologic treatment would be inconsistent with environmental attributions and also may affirm the patient's anxiety of being "crazy" or being seen as crazy. Nonadherence to medication may be rationalized as the result of chemical intolerance to the medication. Relief of psychiatric symptoms by any form of treatment jeopardizes the patient's invalid status. Also, many patients manifesting traits characteristic of certain personality disorders (borderline, narcissistic, antisocial, histrionic) report feeling worse when medications seem objectively to be fostering improvements. It has been suggested that borderline patients may fear abandonment of treatment with improvement or disinhibition of behavioral controls with decreases in depression or anxiety.[61] Also, maintenance of symptoms of depression or anxiety may be associated with primary gain as an avoidance or displacement defense.

WHO IS AT RISK OF ACQUIRING IEI?

In assisting an IEI patient to restructure mistaken beliefs about environmental intolerances it is helpful for the therapist to have an appreciation of why the patient is susceptible to such unsubstantiated thinking and suggestion. The answer often is found in understanding the personality traits of the individual and the psychological defenses used to displace emotional conflict and the resulting symptoms of depression and anxiety. Treatment to ameliorate these symptoms generally is necessary before initiating therapy to restructure mistaken beliefs about IEI.

Personality and Personality Disorders

Personality is defined by complex genetic, personal, and environmental factors, including the perceptual and cognitive processes that describe both the long-standing trait characteristics of the individual, and the phasic physiological state changes associated with the stress-response. Everyday world experiences and percepts derive their personalized meaning from these systems as the individual organizes and plans interactive behavior with the world. Well-adjusted individuals express their personality through effective coping styles. Maladjusted individuals rely on ineffective psychological defenses. Depression, anxiety, phobia, and somatization often are the clinical syndromes that reflect the output of personality disorders.[54] In such cases, the unique meaning of the clinical condition is influenced by traits of personality and personality disorders as well as by psychosocial stressors that define the context of the symptoms. To make matters more complex, a host of psychological defense mechanisms may be employed in various combinations and hierarchies by different individuals.

Patients with personality disorders have **maladaptive and inflexible responses to stress** and do not cope well with the demands of the outside world. Instead, they attempt to make the world adapt to them. Often lacking empathy with others, they consistently fail to see themselves as others see them. Their interpersonal relationships remain perpetually troubled and entangled. They tend to describe their past problematic life experiences and their failure to cope as irrelevant to their present environmental condition. Instead, they externalize their difficulties, and focus on their immediate troubles believed to be caused by those projections. Unfortunately, patients with personality disorders usually are extremely irritating and, consequently, are more scorned than studied and treated.

Several studies of IEI patients identified obsessive-compulsive symptomatology[19,92,85] and personality traits.[72] These patients typically are fluent in arguing the latest toxicogenic theory with conviction. Some eloquently argue the rationalizations for negative medical findings, often parroting what they have been told by an environmental physician or what has been absorbed from publications promoted by advocacy groups. During initial history taking, IEI patients with obsessive-compulsive symptomatology have extensive, well-documented summaries for their complaints and environmental experiences. They usually are quite eager to share their history. Spending enough time with these patients in history taking, physical exam, test interpretation, debriefing challenge testing results, and comparing each patient's reactions to the realities of objective results is necessary to establish a working doctor-patient relationship. When undergoing blinded provocation challenges, negative results that fail to corroborate the patient's hypothesis may not be conclusive to him or her. "Should have, would have, could have" scenarios abound and serve as masterful rebuttal, often unrecognized by physicians as rationalization and other psychologic defenses.

Patients with obsessive-compulsive traits usually do not present aberrant or histrionic behaviors. Their mental status evaluation typically reflects an individual who presents as well oriented, cooperative, appropriately dressed and groomed, and normal in demeanor, speech, and language. However, IEI patients with obsessive-compulsive traits often show flat, nonresponsive, or guarded affect and lack insight into the psychological significance of their symptoms. Typically, these patients deny that present or past psychological conflicts may be contributing to their current symptoms. When review of medical records reveals no prior psychiatric evaluation or treatment, look for physician notes indicating stress, family discord, depression, or anxiety.

Cognitive Styles

Cognitive styles are defined as the manner in which an individual attends, perceives, and generally processes information. For example, some IEI patients are vigilant for odors and other environmental stimuli that they expect will trigger an adverse reaction. Normal bodily sensations and fatigue are perceived as abnormal and amplified into symptoms. Pain thresholds appear to be low, but so are thresholds of suggestibility. If alternative psychological processes can explain their symptoms, they may deny such explanations, choosing instead to focus on information biased to confirm environmental attribution. Overcoming the limitations of this type of cognitive processing is the first goal in treatment, addressed with self-regulation and behavioral therapies to ameliorate symptoms.

Attribution of symptoms and resulting disabilities is on a continuum, ranging from idle curiosity, to hypochondriacal worries for which the patient has insight, to an overvalued idea with absolute conviction reflecting a closed belief system.[43,60] The IEI patient with a closed belief system dissimulates refuting evidence. Negative findings on laboratory tests are dissembled as flawed or lacking in "sensitivity," or reframed emotionally as frustrating to the patient. When confronted, this type of patient often returns to an advocacy support system that reinforces unsubstantiated beliefs, and he or she is lost to appropriate medical and psychological management.

WHY ARE PATIENTS ATTRACTED TO THESE PHENOMENA?

If viewed as a disease, IEI legitimizes withdrawal from responsibility of work, obligation, and interpersonal relations. Like one of its historical predecessors, neurasthenia, IEI sanctions isolation, depression, anxiety, and demoralization. Motivational factors include factitious disorders, malingering, secondary gain, or primary gain. Factitious disorders and malingering usually are seen in IEI patients with comorbid narcissistic, histrionic, antisocial, or obsessive-compulsive personality traits. This type of individual often is involved in claims of worker's compensation or civil litigation.

Secondary gain is defined as an unconscious means of obtaining attention or benefit. Manifestations of secondary gain can occur alone or in combination (Table 3). The psychodynamic tradition defines primary gain as the avoidance of anxiety that would result if an emotional or intrapsychic conflict became conscious. The cognitive-behavioral psychology approach defines primary gain in terms of overload of coping resources (Table 4).

THE PSYCHOLOGICAL APPROACH TO TREATMENT

By nature, psychotherapy directed at a broad spectrum of disorders is eclectic. Psychotherapists may be identified by their schooling, training, practice, and experience, but most still practice according to personal styles,[1] especially when working with difficult patients who do not adhere to standard treatment regimens. No one psychotherapeutic approach has ever been demonstrated to be any better than any other across a wide spectrum of psychological and psychiatric conditions.[38,79] The success of psychotherapies lies in their common features associated with the establishment of trust, empathy, and rapport between patient and doctor.

TABLE 3. Secondary Gain Motivation and Reinforcement

Interpersonal:	
Sympathy, attention	Protection from criticism
Affection from family and friends	Explanation for not trying
Assurance of importance	Avoidance of difficult relations
Rationalization of failure (avoid humiliation)	
Monetary:	
Disability insurance	Medical insurance
Workers' compensation	Tort litigation
Exemption:	
Responsibility	Achievement
Work and employment	Interaction with the outside world
Power:	
Manipulation and control in relationships	Community problems
Employee empowerment	Political cause

TABLE 4.   Factors Associated with Primary Gain

Trauma and resulting posttraumatic stress disorder	Demoralization
Cultural or economic deprivation	Unbearable loss
Social alienation	

Adapted from Frank JD, Frank JB: Persuasion and Healing: A Comparative Study of Psychotherapy, 3rd ed. Baltimore, Johns Hopkins Press, 1991.

The therapeutic approach that this author has found to be effective in the treatment of IEI patients is somewhat hierarchical. It typically begins with physician education and assurance that alternative medical diagnoses have been considered. This is complemented by supportive psychotherapy, self-regulation of symptoms, and cognitive-behavioral treatment, culminating in insight-oriented psychotherapy with those individuals who choose to explore the etiology of their somatization. The specific interventions include explanation of stress-response physiology and learned sensitivity, self-regulation and relaxation training employing biofeedback, noncritical confrontation of unsubstantiated beliefs, and interpretation of the somatization and projection of anxieties. When opportune, explanation of an alternative etiology is explored. This could be a stress disorder resulting from the inability to cope with current or past significant life events or daily stressors. The most severe cases usually have an etiology which originates in disruptions of personality occurring during childhood development as a consequence of childhood abuse and neglect leading to somatization and beliefs of victimization in adulthood.[13,99]

Guidelines for the physician working with somatizing patients[34] also apply to IEI patients,[107] chronic fatigue patients,[53] and patients with other types of functional somatic syndromes[10] (Table 5). In therapy, there is no contesting of the validity of the patient's physical and emotional feelings of distress and suffering; argument usually focuses on the etiology. This author believes that the symptoms and attributions of IEI patients reflect premorbid stress disorders, somatization, and mood or anxiety disorders which frequently are associated with traits of personality disorders. For these patients, IEI represents an overvalued idea, a disorder of belief.

As a therapist, the first question to ask oneself when treating an IEI patient is, "Is it rational to be logical?" Insight-oriented psychotherapy is contraindicated in

TABLE 5.   Physician Guidelines for Difficult Somatizers

1. Establish the significance of psychosocial factors in the patient's illness—use the symptom-oriented, nondirective interview.
2. Maintain an unbiased interest; communicate an air of nonjudgmental concern.
3. Take a complete history and perform a physical examination.
4. "Don't just do something, stand there!" Have the confidence not to order unnecessary diagnostic studies to rule out organic disease.
5. Do not attempt to reassure by stating that the problem is emotional.
6. Accept the symptoms. Respect the adaptive value of the illness.
7. Set up regular visits to develop the therapeutic relationship.
8. Be alert for new developments. Alternative medical diagnoses can develop in the patient who cries wolf.
9. Treatment may be prolonged. Ending a therapeutic relationship can be a difficult task.
10. Be aware of personal attitudes [countertransference].

Adapted from Drossman DA: The problem patient: Evaluation and care of medical patients with psychosocial disturbances. Ann Intern Med 88:366-372, 1978.

many IEI patients, at least initially. Often, behavioral and cognitive-behavioral therapy, stress management, and supportive psychotherapy are the most effective ways to begin treatment. But even before that, the most effective approach is educational[11] (e.g., explaining the physiology and psychophysiology that underlie stress symptoms).[41] Psychophysiological profiling of stress responses also can be used. Brainwave mapping by quantitative electroencephalogram can identify patterns associated with activation or attentional vigilance and help the patient to understand why they may experience attention problems.[97] Meditation or attention training is helpful in mediating EEG biofeedback in individuals who are vigilant for environmental agents or who amplify their body sensations into "reactions."[82] Muscle tension can be seen in the excessive activity on the electromyogram (EMG). Excessive tension in the muscles of the head, neck, and shoulders can be associated with tension headaches and may be reduced with EMG biofeedback or massage. Elevated galvanic skin responses reflect autonomic nervous system activation and may explain associated arousal symptoms.[67] Physiological measurements and psychophysiological explanations are usually nonthreatening to the IEI patient.

In addition, explanations of learned sensitivity, the placebo-response, and the physiology of the stress-response may overcome resistance to addressing other psychosocial factors.[95]

Provocation Challenge Studies

Information from individualized provocation challenge studies adds an invaluable educational and therapeutic tool.[81,98] A state-of-the-art isolation challenge chamber and double-blind, placebo-controlled conditions are not always necessary to test a patient's own hypothesis about environmental sensitivities.[80] Many IEI patients complain of "reactions" to exposures in the ambient environment without any "masking" effects. When a symptom has an objective measurement associated with it, placebo controls are indicated only if the individual can demonstrate a positive response under open provocation challenge.

For example, an open provocation challenge was conducted in a hospital neurodiagnostic laboratory on a middle-aged woman with a 10-year history of disability attributed to chemical sensitivities. She complained that exposure to specific fragrances immediately elicited seizures.[96] The baseline EEG was normal. Immediately after each provocation with air deodorant and perfume, she consistently showed (via video-EEG monitoring) both generalized tonic/clonic and multifocal myoclonic jerking, at times was nonresponsive, spoke with slurred speech, and complained of right-sided paralysis and lethargy. None of these events were associated with EEG abnormalities. The convulsions were a manifestation of psychogenic pseudoseizures which had been iatrogenically reinforced. In this case, the results did not facilitate psychiatric referral. Nevertheless, other patients less vested in malingering and maintaining the sick role may reassess their beliefs and consider psychological explanations and appropriate intervention.

Psychotherapies

The objectives for different types of psychologic or psychiatric interventions are orchestrated according to the patient's goals and needs as well as the availability of cognitive and emotional resources (Table 6). Short-term therapies can help the patient establish a sense of being in control and able to cope with stress (Table 7). As therapy progresses and rapport develops, the truth of the belief system can be broached. A practical guide for using cognitive-behavioral techniques with patients

TABLE 6. Psychotherapeutic Objectives and Approaches

Controlling symptoms: stress management, psychophysiological self-regulation, psychotropic medication

Changing behavior/belief: behavior modification (systematic desensitization), cognitive-behavioral therapy (cognitive distortions)

Getting at the underlying issues: cognitive, insight-oriented psychotherapy

who have functional somatic symptoms is available.[87] A postulate commonly shared by cognitive-behavior therapists and cognitive therapists from psychodynamic schools is that affect, sensory reactions, and motor responses are associated with beliefs operant in the interpretation of an experience. It may be helpful to present and interpret common cognitive distortions seen in depression and other disorders (Table 8).[15] Traditional insight-oriented or psychodynamic psychotherapy may best be withheld until the patient is ready to process the underlying conflicts and realizes that the mistaken beliefs about the effects of environmental exposures are irrelevant to the etiology of the symptoms (Table 9).

The limits of **behavioral desensitization treatment** of phobic avoidance were noted in a study of three IEI patients.[46] By the end of treatment, all three patients had acquired significant relaxation skills and were able to sustain prolonged exposure to a wide array of noxious chemicals without demonstrating physiological or symptomatic activation. However, these effects were sustained in only one of the three patients upon follow-up. This patient was the only one who was not under the care of an environmental physician.

While cognitive-behavioral and cognitive psychotherapies are considered the treatments of choice for functional somatic syndromes,[10] there are limitations. The psychotherapies presuppose that the patient is open to rational discussion of cognitive distortions and unsubstantiated beliefs. Also, the patient must demonstrate the capacity for insight, at least to the extent of recognizing that the cognitive distortions lead to irrational beliefs as well as depression and anxiety, which in turn may exacerbate the somatization.

For traumatized patients who suffer the sequelae of posttraumatic stress disorder, especially those with a history of childhood abuse and emotional deprivation, it is important to offer a safe environment in therapy for them to reconstruct deeply wounding and humiliating experiences for which they may continue to feel in some way responsible.[23] The more the memory of the trauma can be reevaluated and contained in the context of the past, the less frightening the effects are in the present, where they are displaced onto the physical environment. Reduced fear and terror allow the giving up of false defenses. One sign of a successful therapy is that the re-

TABLE 7. Guidelines for Short-Term Psychotherapy

Confidence: To facilitate confidence in the technique, begin with an elaborated, well planned rationale that provides an initial structure.

Relevance: Provide training in meaningful skills that the patient can use to feel more effective in handling daily life.

Genealization: Emphasize independent use of these skills outside of the therapist's office.

Success and reinforcement: The training should provide enough structure and explanation so that the skill can be mastered in the office and generalized to at least some real world situations.

Self-reliance: Encourage the patient's attribution that improvement is caused by the patient's increased skillfulness, not by the therapist's skillfulness or the magical aspects of a therapeutic ritual.

TABLE 8.   Common Cognitive Distortions

Dichotomous thinking	Undergeneralization
Selective abstraction	Catastrophizing
Arbitrary inference	Decatastrophizing
Circular logic	Misattributed causality
Overgeneralization	Rationalization of lies

Adapted from Beck AT: Cognitive Therapy and Emotional Disorders. New York, International Universities Press, 1976.

structured knowledge about reality displaces the patient's original distortions and overvalued ideas about environmental intolerances. The sometimes unexpected lack of resistance that may be encountered by the therapist during this process should not be surprising, since an effective coping mechanism serves the patient better than a false defense. Ultimately, the test of any psychotherapy is whether the patient can learn to ameliorate debilitating symptoms, mitigate past fears, and maintain effective coping behaviors in daily life.

A Model for Anxiety and Panic Disorder

The complexity of treating IEI patients is captured in a treatment model of panic disorder developed by Shear and associates. It integrates psychodynamic, neurophysiological, and cognitive-behavioral theoretical formulations and clinical approaches, and emphasizes the importance of early childhood experiences of trauma and emotional deprivation.[27,88,89] In a controlled study, patients with anxiety disorder had significantly higher incidence of history of childhood physical and sexual abuse than a community sample, with a particular association between sexual abuse and panic disorder in women.[103]

The model was illustrated with observations on nine (6 females, 3 males) patients who had panic attacks.[89] In the initial interview, all nine patients denied having anxiety prior to the onset of the panic attacks. They also believed that stress was unrelated to the onset of panic. Later in the interview, stressors and significant life events were identified which preceded the onset of panic attacks, a finding consistent with other studies.[66,74] Heightened frustration and resentment with relationships, social relations, and employment characterized these types of stressful events. The following case reads like a vignette of an IEI patient, were "environmental reaction" substituted for panic episode:

> *One patient initially disavowed being nervous or anxious before the onset of panic [environmental reaction]. However, later in the interview, she*

TABLE 9.   Four Principles of Psychodynamic Treatment

1. During treatment, unconscious (inhibited) material becomes conscious.
2. The mobilization of unconscious material is achieved mainly through the interpretation of information presented during free association and the patient's emotional interpersonal experience (transference).
3. The patient resists recognition of unconscious content.
4. Through the transference relation with the therapist, resistance is overcome, and childhood experiences are reenacted to provide insight and resolution.

Adapted from Alexander F: The dynamics of psychotherapy in the light of learning theory. Am J Psychiatry 120:440-448, 1963.

explained that although she never thought of herself as an anxious person, other people said she was. She noted that she had always been "claustrophobic" in situations such as traffic jams or department stores, where she would become anxious and feel that she was trapped. She further described herself as a "worrier, always thinking the worst." The patient initially stressed that things were fine before her first panic episode [environmental reaction]. However, in the course of the interview she revealed that she was chronically unhappy at her job, where she felt unfairly treated—overworked, underpaid, and emotionally drained. She described her boyfriend of 3 years as "very cold." She felt shortchanged by him and often felt hurt and useless. She finally said, "I think that was one of the reasons I got so nervous."[89]

Like this panic patient, many IEI patients reveal stressful life events and experiences of frustration and anxiety after establishing rapport with a doctor or psychotherapist. These patients frequently are more amenable to referral for stress management treatment and have a good prognosis. Treatment of patients with closed belief systems, who are well defended by denial of psychological factors in their lives and often are involved in litigation, may require examination of prior medical and psychological records to unearth evidence of emotional disorders, stressful life events, and poor relationships. A commonality between panic and IEI patients is that the origin of the anxiety that manifests as panic attacks *precedes* the alleged event of onset, often dating to childhood trauma or neglect.

Of the nine panic patients interviewed by Shear, all described at least one parent as angry and frightening, critical, or controlling. Discomfort with aggression in adulthood emerged as a theme in seven patients. Each patient complained about aspects of a relationship or job situation and indicated having chronic feelings of resentment and a sense of injustice. However, in each case the patient felt too guilty or anxious to confront the situation, fears that imply an earlier etiology. Seven patients described feelings of low self-esteem or prominent negative self-attributes. Complaints and aggressive feelings were regularly accompanied by contradictory comments. For example, one patient described her family as very tense but quickly added that they were close and loving. Such neurotic symptoms are best explained by predisposing personality factors:

The interviews revealed themes of early life anxiety and shyness, unsupportive parental relationships, and a chronic sense of being trapped and troubled by frustration and resentment. Each patient described frightening, controlling, or critical parents and most described feelings of inadequacy and/or self reproach. Aggression was prominent, uncomfortable, and often managed with efforts to contradict complaints and/or turn negative into positive attributes. This consistency was impressive and led the interviewers to revise their view that the pathogenic mechanism of panic was primarily physiological.[89]

Psychotropic Medications

While IEI patients have been described to be depressed, their symptoms are not of the type that usually remit with a course of antidepressant medication. It is an oversimplification to suggest that these patients are "just suffering from depression." Many patients appear to have biological and psychodynamic correlates analogous to individuals suffering from post-traumatic stress disorder (PTSD) arising from childhood traumas. Note that these traumas are premorbid to environmental exposures believed to result in chemical sensitivities. The effects of PTSD are distinct from clinical depression,[67,112] and some symptoms may be exacerbated by antidepressant medications. Furthermore, most IEI patients refuse medication or fail to adhere to them if prescribed.

There may be a tacit bias among some psychiatrists to diagnose only conditions for which there is a pharmacologic treatment, most often depression and anxiety.[39] Existing assessment procedures are biased to categorize multisystem somatic complaints as symptoms of depression and anxiety.[40] This bias may arise, in part, because somatoform disorders are considered among the most difficult to treat and generally have poor prognosis.[37,68] Antidepressant medications in general have been found effective in some studies of functional somatic syndromes.[48] However, selective serotonin reuptake inhibitors (SSRIs; e.g., Prozac, Zoloft, Paxil) also have been shown to be ineffective in some studies of chronic fatigue syndrome[52,105] and fibromyalgia.[111]

Negative health perception is characteristic of patients with a history of childhood sexual abuse. In a review of seven studies from demographically diverse populations, controlling for depression did not remove patients' self negative perceptions of their health.[42] Nevertheless, appropriate medication can facilitate an emotional state that helps the patient participate effectively in psychotherapy. The psychotherapeutic art with IEI patients involves reducing their concerns about sensitivity to medications and convincing them that they could benefit.

A Case Example

The complexity of therapeutic techniques is illustrated in the following IEI case presentation of an individual who showed lack of psychodynamic insight.[84] Upon beginning therapy, the patient professed intolerance for his luxurious home, his cars, the company of his wife, and any form of travel. He lived alone in an old, downtown motel room, the only environment he perceived as safe. Among the many chemical agents to which he reported intolerance, he expressed particular sensitivity to the odor of rubbing alcohol. Behavioral systematic desensitization was employed only after months of twice weekly psychotherapy in which a therapeutic alliance was established. The patient mastered self-regulation skills, using biofeedback for symptom regulation, before the systematic desensitization procedure was initiated.

Restructuring of the IEI belief was underway by educating the patient to the shortcomings of the unsubstantiated theories and practices of clinical ecology. He had undergone removal and replacement of all his dental amalgams at the hands of a Colorado dentist who since has lost his license to practice. The patient came to realize that heavy metal was not affecting the magnetic polarity in his brain. Cognitive therapy techniques were employed to identify and analyze cognitive distortions and inconsistencies in his logic. Antidepressant medication was prescribed for symptoms of extreme fatigue and attentional problems associated with depression, with good therapeutic response.

Interestingly, the systematic sensitization may well have been the ritual that effectively gave him an acceptable explanation as to why he was no longer reacting to the odor of alcohol.

> *A not infrequently and easily overlooked function of therapeutic rituals is to provide a face-saving way for a patient to abandon a symptom or complaint without admitting that it was trivial or produced for some ulterior motive.*[38]

The tolerance for the odor of alcohol generalized to his other perceived chemical sensitivities. Shortly thereafter, he traveled throughout Europe.

Unfortunately, IEI recurred several years later, after the publication of our 1992 report. He was involved in a motor vehicle accident in which his wife was severely injured. Initially, she was in critical condition from internal injuries; she survived, but had a residue of debilitating chronic pain. The anxiety of almost losing his wife followed by her disability led him to project his anxiety onto the environment. A year after the accident, he was again referred for additional therapy. He was unaware that he was experiencing symptoms of anxiety and depression. He had again tried a variety of unsubstantiated treatments including exotic teas and supplements, none of which worked for him. With the aid of cognitive-behavioral approaches, he came to more realistic appraisals and attributions of his symptoms. After several months of treatment, he appeared less anxious and recognized that his alleged environmental reactions were inconsistent. Whereas he complained of symptoms with trivial chemical detections, he could attend and tolerate large dinners, concerts, and other public gatherings where he had a multitude of chemical encounters. His wife had also recovered to the degree that she could travel again. It is possible that her becoming less accommodating of his somatization had something to do with his recovery.

WHO MAY BENEFIT FROM TREATMENT

In general, somatizing patients who have a strong belief in a physical explanation for their symptoms have a poor prognosis.[43,109] IEI patients who remain enmeshed in the advocacy networks and continue to be treated by environmental medicine physicians are poor candidates for psychotherapy and also are at risk to become more psychologically disabled.[94]

Recently, federal and state insurance legislation has granted "parity for mental disorders." But parity in this legal context is narrowly interpreted to include disorders generally believed to have a biological basis, such as major psychoses (schizophrenia), affective disorders (depression, bipolar affective disorder), and some anxiety disorders (panic disorder and obsessive-compulsive disorder), which have corresponding medication regimens in the biological psychiatrist's treatment model. Disorders that do not respond well to medications and require comprehensive, long-term psychotherapy, such as PTSD, somatoform disorders, and personality disorders, are excluded from parity. This seems to be poor risk-management for somatizing patients,[9] especially for IEI patients with an overvalued idea about chemical intolerances.

As a therapeutic alliance is established, the bridge to traditional insight-oriented cognitive psychotherapy[6,7] can be crossed with many IEI patients, even some who are the most difficult to treat. Clinical experience suggests that these are the patients who reported histories of traumatic and chronic childhood abuse or neglect.[76] For many IEI patients who have been able to process their childhood traumas in therapy, the emotionally disruptive sequelae have become manageable.[99]

Clinical cases of improvement have been reported for various disorders characterized by somatization and mistaken beliefs of a physical cause, using a variety of therapeutic interventions in inpatient[51,82] and outpatient settings.[4,28,32,99,109] These approaches also have been effective in the treatment of patients without physical attributions for functional somatic pain symptoms such as chronic pain,[16] irritable bowel syndrome,[49] childhood trauma,[64] and phobia and hypochondria.[106] Patients who recover or show improvement after appropriate psychologic or psychiatric treatment are evidence against the toxicogenic theory that psychiatric symptoms were primarily determined or exacerbated by environmental intolerances and the resulting disabilities.

CONCLUSION

Throughout what may be a lengthy therapy, it is important to demonstrate understanding and empathy for the IEI patient's distress. For the therapist, patience is paramount because healing often requires waiting for the patient to find an exit out of their world of mistaken beliefs and ritualistic practice of unsubstantiated treatments. Entering into a world resembling reality often is threatening to an individual who has relied on psychological defenses to deny, displace, or distort a personal history of distress and trauma that created feelings of anxiety, helplessness, and/or despair. The therapist can only guide the patient along this precarious and painful journey, accepting that ultimately the outcome is the patient's choosing. The patient cannot be rescued from this journey, nor be transported to the real world by the proclamation that his or her beliefs about IEI are scientifically unproved.

Ideally, psychotherapy begins with assessing the patient's possible world, including knowledge, beliefs, emotions, sensations, personality traits, defenses and coping mechanisms, self-image, and the perceptions of the individuals with whom the person interacts. Progressively, but in no particular order, the patient discloses fear and terror, anger and rage, pain and suffering, or depression and anxiety. In therapy these feelings and issues are ameliorated or resolved, and beliefs about the world are aligned with reality. For such a radical shift to occur, the patient must relinquish the sick role and displaced feelings of victimization.

This author frequently is asked, "How do you treat IEI?" The person asking the question usually anticipates one specific approach or technique. However, any psychotherapy that facilitates rapport and gives the patient confidence that he or she may be helped, addresses the underlying personality issues that manifest as somatization, and—especially—offers the opportunity for the patient to explore traumatic childhood experiences is of value. Anything less is unlikely to help the more severely disturbed IEI patients.

Even in a successful therapy, the ideal outcome of complete wellness is rarely, if ever, fully achieved with difficult patients. Hopefully, the approach I have outlined provides some useful heuristics for setting therapeutic goals, planning intervention strategies, and applying behavioral and cognitive methods. These suggestions are no more than that, and should not be taken as definitive. After all, clinical experience has taught us that no two therapists practice alike, and that no particular form of psychotherapy is generally more effective than any other. Irrespective of the kind of psychotherapy practiced, the common objective is to restructure the knowledge of the patient toward a more positive concept of self, a more realistic appraisal of the physical-environment, and a less frightening interpretation of the person-environment.

The most difficult task for the doctor is to transfer the patient onto the path of psychotherapy. Subsequent steps include guiding the individual on his or her journey and finding the means by which the patient can feel self-confident, accept self-reliance, and learn new coping skills to replace the psychological defense mechanisms which, in fact, never resolved conflicts and anxieties. This journey is made even more difficult by the obstacles placed by environmental physicians who prescribe unsubstantiated treatments based on scientifically unfounded toxicogenic theories to exploit the vulnerabilities of patients.

REFERENCES

1. Alexander F: The dynamics of psychotherapy in the light of learning theory. Am J Psychiatry 120:440–448, 1963.
2. Altenkirch H, Hopmann D, Brockmeier B, Walter G: Neurological investigations in 23 cases of pyrethroid intoxication reported to the German Federal Health Office. Neurotoxicology 17:645–652, 1996.
3. American Academy of Allergy Asthma and Immunology Board of Directors: Position statement: idiopathic environmental intolerances. J Allergy Clin Immunol 103:36–40, 1999.
4. Andersson B, Berg M, Arnetz BB, Melin L, Langlet I, Liden S: A cognitive-behavioral treatment of patients suffering from "electric hypersensitivity." J Occup Environ Med 38:752–758, 1996.
5. Bardana, EJ: Sick building syndrome-a wolf in sheep's clothing. Ann Allergy Asthma Immunol 79:283–94, 1997.
6. Barnett J: Insight and therapeutic change. Contemp Psychoanalysis 14:534–544, 1978.
7. Barnett J: Cognitive repair in the treatment of the neuroses. J Am Acad Psychoanalysis 8:39–55, 1980.
8. Barsky AJ: Patients who amplify bodily sensations. Ann Int Med 91:63–70, 1979.
9. Barsky AJ, Borus JF: Somatization and Medicalization in the era of managed care. JAMA 274(24):1931–1934, 1995.
10. Barsky AJ, Borus JF: Functional somatic syndromes. Ann Intern Med 130:910–921, 1999.
11. Barsky AJ, Geringer E, Wool CA: A cognitive-educational treatment for hypochondriasis. Gen Hosp Psychiatry 10:322–327, 1988.
12. Barsky AJ, Klerman GL: Overview: hypochondriasis, bodily complaints, and somatic styles. Am J Psychiatry 140:273–283, 1983.
13. Barsky AJ, Wool C, Barnett MC, Cleary PD: Histories of childhood trauma in adult hypochondriacal patients. Am J Psychoanalysis 151:397–401, 1994.
14. Bass C, Benjamin S: The management of chronic somatization. Bri J Psychiatry 162:472–480, 1993.
15. Beck AT: Cognitive Therapy and the Emotional Disorders. New York, International Universities Press, 1976.
16. Benjamin S: Psychological treatment of chronic pain: a selective review. J Psychosom Res 33:121–131, 1989.
17. Binkley KE, Kutcher S: Panic response to sodium lactate infusion in patients with multiple chemical sensitivity syndrome. J Allergy Clin Immunol 99:570–574, 1997.
18. Black DW: Iatrogenic (physician-induced) hypochondriasis: Four patient examples of "chemical sensitivity." Psychosomatics 37:390–393, 1996.
19. Black DW, Rathe A, Goldstein RB: Environmental illness: A controlled study of 26 subjects with `20th century disease.' JAMA 264:3166–3170, 1990.
20. Black DW, Rathe A, Goldstein RB: Measures of distress in 26 "environmentally ill" subjects. Psychosomatics 34:131–138, 1993.
21. Bolla KI: Neurobehavioral performance in multiple chemical sensitivities. Reg Toxicol Pharmacol 24:S52–S54, 1996.
22. Boss LP:Epidemic hysteria: a review of the published literature. Epidemiol Rev 19(2):233–243, 1997.
23. Brewin CR, Andrews B, Gotlib IH: Psychopathology and early experience: A reappraisal of retrospective reports. Psychol Bull 113:82–98, 1993.
24. Brodsky CM: 'Allergic to everything': A medical subculture. Psychosomatics 24(8):731–742, 1983.
25. Brodsky CM: The psychiatric epidemic in the American workplace. Occup Med State Art Rev 3:653–662, 1988.
26. Burton R: The anatomy of melancholy. London:Longman, Rees & Co., 1837. (Originally published in 1621).
27. Busch FN, Cooper AM, Klerman GL, Penzer RJ, Shapiro T, Shear MK: Neurophysiological, cognitive-behavioral, and psychoanalytic approaches to panic disorder: toward an integration. Psychoanalytic Inquiry 11:316–332, 1991.
28. Butler S, Chalder T, Ron M, Wessely S: Cognitive therapy in chronic fatigue syndrome. J Neurol Neurosurg Psychiatry 54:153–158, 1991.
29. Chrousos GP, McCarty R, Pacak K, Cizza G, Sternberg E, Gold PW, Kvetnansky R (eds.): Stress: Basis Mechanisms and Clinical Implications. Ann NY Acad Sci, vol. 771, 1995.
30. Chrousos GP, Gold PW: The concepts of stress and stress system disorders: Overview of physical and behavioral homeostasis. JAMA 267:1244–1252, 1992.
31. Colligan MJ, Pennebaker JW, Murphy LR (eds): Mass Psychogenic Illness: A Social Psychological Analysis. Hillsdale, NJ, Erlbaum, 1982.

32. Deale A, Chalder T, Marks I, Wessely S: Cognitive behavior therapy for chronic fatigue syndrome: a randomized controlled trial. Am J Psychiatry 154:408–414, 1997.
33. Deary IJ: A taxonomy of medically unexplained symptoms. J Psychosom Res 47(1):51–59, 1999.
34. Drossman DA: The problem patient: Evaluation and care of medical patients with psychosocial disturbances. Ann Int Med 88:366–372, 1978.
35. Ellis, E. Clinical ecology: Myth and Reality. Buffalo Physician 1986;19(5):23–28.
36. Fiedler N, Kipen, HM, Deluca J, McNeil K, Natelson B: A controlled comparison of multiple chemical sensitivities and chronic fatigue syndrome. Psychosom Med 58:38–49, 1996.
37. Ford CV: Somatization and fashionable diagnoses: illness as a way of life. Scand J Work Environ Health 23 suppl 3:7–16, 1997.
38. Frank JD, Frank JB: Persuasion and Healing: A Comparative Study of Psychotherapy, 3rd ed. Baltimore, Johns Hopkins Press, 1991.
39. Goldberg D: A dimensional model for common mental disorders. Bri J Psychiatry 168(suppl. 30):44–49, 1996.
40. Goldberg D, Bridges K: Minor psychiatric disorders and neurasthenia in general practice. In Gastpar M, Kielholz P (eds.), Problems of Psychiatry in General Practice. Lewiston, NY, Hogrefe & Huber Publishers, 1991, pp. 79–88.
41. Goldberg D, Gask L, O'Dowd T: The treatment of somatization: teaching techniques of re-attribution. J Psychosom Res 33:689–695, 1989.
42. Golding JM, Cooper ML, George LK: Sexual assault history and health perceptions: seven general population studies. Health Psychology 16:417–425, 1997.
43. Gomez R, Schvaneveldt RW, Staudenmayer H: Assessing beliefs about `environmental illness/multiple chemical sensitivity.' J Health Psychol 1:107–123, 1996.
44. Gothe CJ, Molin CM, Nilsson CG. The environmental somatization syndrome. Psychosomatics 36(1):1–11, 1995.
45. Gots, RE: Medical hypothesis and medical practice: autointoxication and multiple chemical sensitivities. Reg Toxicol Pharmacol 18:61–78, 1993.
46. Guglielmi RS, Cox DJ, Spyker DA: Behavioral treatment of phobic avoidance in multiple chemical sensitivity. J Behav Therapy Exp Psychiatry 25:197–209, 1994.
47. Gupta, K, Perharic L, Volans GN, Murray VSG, Watson JP: Apparent poisoning by wood preservatives: an attributional syndrome. J Psychosom Res 43:391–398, 1997.
48. Gruber A, Hudson J, Pope H: The management of treatment resistant depression in disorders of the interface of psychiatry and medicine: fibromyalgia, chronic fatigue syndrome, migraine, irritable bowel syndrome, atypical facial pain, and premenstrual dysphoric disorder. Psychiat Clin North Am 19:351–369, 1996.
49. Guthrie E, Creed F, Dawson D, Tomenson, B: A controlled trial of psychological treatment for the irritable bowel syndrome. Gastroenterol 100:450–457, 1991.
50. Hahn M, Bonkovsky HL: Multiple chemical sensitivity syndrome and porphyria. Arch Int Med 157:281–285, 1997.
51. Haller E: Successful management of patients with "multiple chemical sensitivity" on an inpatient psychiatric unit. J Clin Psychiatry 54:196–199, 1993.
52. Hickie I, Wilson A: A catecholamine model of fatigue. Bri J Psychiatry 165:275–276, 1994.
53. Howard LM, Wessely S: Psychiatry in the allergy clinic: the nature and management of patients with non-allergic symptoms. Clin Exp Allergy 25:503–513, 1995.
54. Hudziak JJ, Boffeli TJ, Kriesman JJ, Battaglia MM, Stanger C, Guze SB: Clinical study of the relation of borderline personality disorder to Briquet's syndrome (hysteria), somatization disorder, antisocial personality disorder, and substance abuse disorders. Am J Psychiatry 153:1598–1606, 1996.
55. Katon W, Kleinman A, Rosen G: Depression and somatization: A review Part I. Am J Med 72:127–35, 1992.
56. Katon W, Kleinman A, Rosen G: Depression and somatization: A review Part II. Am J Med 72:241–247, 1992.
57. Kellner, R. Somatization--theories and research. J Nerv Ment Dis 178:150–160, 1990.
58. Kroenke K, Koslowe P, Roy M: Symptoms in 18,495 Persian Gulf War veterans. J Occup Environ Med 40:520–528.
59. Leznoff A: Provocative challenges in patients with multiple chemical sensitivity. J Allergy Clin Immunol 99:438–442, 1997.
60. McKenna PJ: Disorders with overvalued ideas. Bri J Psychiatry 145:579–585, 1984.
61. Millon T: Disorders of Personality DSM-IV and Beyond. 2nd ed. New York, Wiley, 1996, p. 689.
62. Ooi PL, Goh, KT: Sick building syndrome: an emerging stress-related disorder. Intl J Epi 26:1243–1249, 1997.

63. Pearson DJ, Rix KJB, Bentley SJ: Food allergy: How much in the mind? A clinical and psychiatric study of suspected food hypersensitivity. Lancet June:1259–1261, 1983.
64. Pennebaker JW, Susman JR: Disclosure of traumas and psychosomatic processes. Soc Sci Med 26:327–332, 1988.
65. Pennebaker JW, Watson D: The psychology of somatic symptoms. In Kirmayer LJ, Robbins JM (eds.): Current Concepts of Somatization: Research and Clinical Perspectives. Washington, DC, American Psychiatric Press, 1991, pp. 21–35.
66. Pollard CA, Pollard HJ, Corn KJ: Panic onset and mayor life events in the lives of agoraphobics: A test of contiguity. J Abnorm Psychol 98:318–321, 1989.
67. Prins A, Kaloupec DG, Keane TM: Psychophysiological evidence for autonomic arousal and startle in traumatized adult populations. In Friedman MJ, Charney DS, Deutch AY (eds): Neurobiological and Clinical consequences of Stress: From Normal Adaptation to PTSD. Philadelphia, Lippincott-Raven Publishers, 1995, pp. 291–314.
68. Quill TE: Somatization Disorder: One of medicine's blind spots. JAMA 254(21):3075–3079, 1985.
69. Randolph DC, Ranavaya MI, Cocchiarella L, Klimek E, Beller TA: Multiple chemical sensitivity syndrome: impairment and disability issues. American Academy of Disability Evaluating Physicians Position Paper. Disability 8 suppl:1–10, 1999.
70. Rix KJB, Pearson DJ, Bentley SJ: A psychiatric study of patients with supposed food allergy. Bri J Psychiatry 145:121–126, 1984.
71. Robbins JM, Kirmayer LJ, Kapusta MA: Illness worry and disability in fibromyalgia syndrome. Intl J Psychiatry Med 20:49–63, 1990.
72. Rosenberg SJ, Freedman MR, Schmaling KG, Rose C: Personality styles of patients asserting environmental illness. J Occup Med 32:678–681, 1990.
73. Ross PM, Whysner J, Covello VT, Kuschner M, Rifkind AB, Sedler MJ, Trichopoulos D, Williams GM. Olfaction and symptoms in multiple chemical sensitivities syndrome. Prevent Med 28:467–480, 1999.
74. Roy-Byrne PP, Geraci M, Uhde TW: Life events and onset of panic disorder. Am J Psychiatry 143:1424–1427, 1986.
75. Sapolsky RM: Stress, the Aging Brain, and the Mechanisms of Neuron Death. Cambridge, MA, MIT Press, 1992.
76. Saporta JAJr, Gans JS: Taking a history of childhood trauma in psychotherapy. J Psychotherapy Prac Res 4:194–204, 1995.
77. Schottenfeld RS: Workers with multiple chemical sensitivities: A psychiatric approach to diagnosis and treatment. Occup Med State Art Rev 2:739–753, 1987.
78. Schweitzer R, Robertson DL, Kelly B, Whiting J: Illness behaviour of patients with chronic fatigue syndrome. J Psychosom Res 38:41–49, 1993.
79. Seligman MEP: The effectiveness of psychotherapy: the Consumer Reports study. Am Psychologist 50:965–974, 1995.
80. Selner JC: Chamber challenges: the necessity of objective observation. Reg Toxicol Pharmacol 24:S87–S95, 1996.
81. Selner JC, Staudenmayer H: The practical approach to the evaluation of suspected environmental exposures: Chemical intolerance. Ann Allergy 55(5):665–673, 1985.
82. Selner JC, Staudenmayer, H: The relationship of the environment and food to allergic and psychiatric illness. In Young SH, Rubin JM, Daman HR (eds.): Psychophysiological Aspects of Allergic Disorders. New York, Praeger, 1986, pp. 102–146.
83. Selner JC, Staudenmayer H: Food allergy: psychological considerations. In Metcalfe DD, Sampson HA, Simon RA (eds.), Food Allergy: Adverse Reactions to Foods and Food Additives. Boston, Blackwell Scientific Publications, 1991, pp. 370–381.
84. Selner JC, Staudenmayer H: Psychological factors complicating the diagnosis of work-related chemical illness. Immunol Allergy Clin North Am 12:909–919, 1992.
85. Selner JC, Staudenmayer H: Neuropsychophysiologic observations in patients presenting with environmental illness. Toxicol Ind Health 8:145–155, 1992.
86. Selner JC, Staudenmayer H, Koepke JW, Harvey R, Christopher K: Vocal cord dysfunction: the importance of psychologic factors and provocation challenge testing. J Allergy Clin Immunol 79:726–733, 1987.
87. Sharpe M, Peveler R, Mayou R: The psychological treatment of patients with functional somatic symptoms: a practical guide. J Psychosom Res 36:515–529, 1992.
88. Shear MK: Factors in the etiology and pathogenesis of panic disorder: revisiting the attachment-separation paradigm. Am J Psychiatry 153:125–136, 1996.
89. Shear MK, Cooper AM, Klerman GL, Busch FN, Shapiro T: A psychodynamic model of panic disorder. Am J Psychiatry 150:859–866, 1993.

90. Shorter E: From Paralysis to Fatigue: A History of Psychosomatic Illness in the Modern Era. New York, Free Press/Macmillan, 1992.
91. Shorter E: Multiple chemical sensitivity: pseudoscience in historical perspective. Scand J Work Environ Health 23 suppl 3:35–42, 1997.
92. Simon GE, Daniell W, Stockbridge H, Claypoole K, Rosenstock L: Immunologic, psychological and neuropsychological factors in multiple chemical sensitivity. Ann Int Med 19:97–103, 1993.
93. Simon GE, Katon WJ, Sparks PJ: Allergic to life: Psychological factors in environmental illness. Am J Psychiatry 147:901–906, 1990.
94. Staudenmayer H: Clinical consequences of the EI/MCS "diagnosis": two paths. Regul Toxicol Pharmacol 24:S96–S110, 1996.
95. Staudenmayer H: Environmental Illness: Myth and Reality. Boca Raton FL, CRC/Lewis, 1999.
96. Staudenmayer H, Kramer R: Psychogenic chemical sensitivity: psychogenic pseudoseizures elicited by provocation challenges with fragrances. J Psychosom Res 47(2):185–190,1999.
97. Staudenmayer H, Selner JC: Neuropsychophysiology during relaxation in generalized, universal 'allergic' reactivity to the environment: A comparison study. J Psychosom Res 34:259–270, 1990.
98. Staudenmayer H, Selner JC, Buhr M: Double-blind provocation challenges in 20 patients present-ing with 'multiple chemical sensitivity.' Regul Pharmacol Toxicol 18:44–53, 1993.
99. Staudenmayer H, Selner ME, Selner JC: Adult sequelae of childhood abuse presenting as environ-mental illness. Ann Allergy 71(6):538–546, 1993.
100. Stewart DE: The changing faces of somatization. Psychosomatics 31(2):153–158, 1990.
101. Stewart, D. E., Raskin, J. Psychiatric assessment of patients with "20th century disease" ("total al-lergy syndrome"). Can Med Assoc J 133:1001–1006, 1985.
102. Terr AI: Clinical ecology in the workplace. J Occup Med 31:257–261, 1989.
103. Stein MB, Walker JR, Anderson G, Hazen AL, Ross CA, Eldridge G, Forde DR: Childhood physi-cal and sexual abuse in patients with anxiety disorders and in a community sample. Am J Psychiatry 153:275–277, 1996.
104. Thomas JG: A critical analysis of multiple chemical sensitivities. Med Hypotheses 50:303–311, 1998.
105. Vercoulen J, Swanink C, Zitman F, Vreden S, Hoofs M, Fennis J, Galama J, van der Meer J, Bleijenberg G: Randomized, double-blind, placebo-controlled study of fluoxetine in chronic fa-tigue syndrome. Lancet 347:858–861, 1996.
106. Warwick HMC, Marks IM: Behavioral treatment of illness phobia and hypochondriasis. Bri J Psychiatry 152:239–241, 1988.
107. Weaver VM: Medical management of the multiple chemical sensitivity patient. Reg Toxicol Pharmacol 24:S111–S115, 1996.
108. Wessely S: Chronic fatigue syndrome: a 20th century illness. Scand J Work Environ Health 23 suppl.3:17–34, 1997.
109. Wilson A, Hickie I, Lloyd A, Hadzi-Pavlovic D, Boughton C, Dwyer J, Wakefield D: Longitudinal study of outcome of chronic fatigue syndrome. BMJ 308:756–759, 1994.
110. Witorsch P, Ayesu K, Balter NJ, Schwartz SL: Multiple chemical sensitivity: clinical features & causal analysis in 61 cases. Presented at the North American Congress of Clinical Toxicology Annual Meeting, Rochester, NY, September 17, 1995.
111. Wolfe F, Cathey MA, Hawley DJ: A double-blind placebo-controlled trial of fluoxetine in fi-bromyalgia. Scand J Rheumatol 23:255-259, 1994.
112. Yehuda R, McFarlane AC: Psychobiology of Posttraumatic Stress Disorder. Ann NY Acad Sci vol. 821, 1997.

CLIFFORD S. MITCHELL, MS, MD, MPH
ALBERT DONNAY, MHS
DONALD R. HOOVER, PhD
JOSEPH B. MARGOLICK, MD, PhD

IMMUNOLOGIC PARAMETERS OF MULTIPLE CHEMICAL SENSITIVITY

From Johns Hopkins School of
  Hygiene and Public Health
Baltimore, Maryland
  and
MCS Referral and Resources
Baltimore, Maryland
  and
Rutgers, the State University of
  New Jersey
Piscataway, New Jersey

Reprint requests to:
Clifford S. Mitchell, MS, MD, MPH
Division of Occupational and
  Environmental Health
Johns Hopkins School of Hygiene
  and Public Health
615 North Wolfe Street,
  Room 7041
Baltimore, MD 21205

From the earliest days in which environmental intolerance to chemicals, or multiple chemical sensitivity (MCS)* was described, etiologic theories have focused on alterations of immune function as a possible mechanism. Levin and Byers reviewed immunologic abnormalities in MCS patients in 1987 and suggested there was an underlying problem with immune regulation, proposing three possible mechanisms—free radical generation, alternation of structural proteins causing autoantibody formation, and hapten-carrier formation.[2] Sparks et al. noted that immunologic theories have been consistently proposed to explain MCS symptoms.[3] Among these are alterations in specific lymphocyte subsets, release of cytokines, or autoantibodies to specific tissues or chemicals. Other theories, such as that of toxicant-induced loss of tolerance (TILT), suggest the involvement of the immune system but do not

---

* In this chapter, we have elected to use the term "multiple chemical sensitivity," rather than "idiopathic environmental intolerance." We have done so in order to maintain consistency with most of the literature cited, particularly clinical studies including our own research in which the case definition used in selecting subjects was similar to Cullen's definition of MCS[1]: the presence of symptomatic responses in several organ systems following exposure to low-levels of multiple chemicals. We do not, by the use of the term MCS, mean to argue for or against any particular theory of causation (including an immunologic cause). Nor do we deny the importance of clarifying what, if any, role chemicals may play in the syndrome. Ultimately, if the cause or causes of this syndrome can be clarified, it will be possible to use more precise terminology.

posit a specific immunologic pathway or mechanism by which patients lose tolerance.[4] However, no one theory has satisfactorily explained all of the presentations or symptoms of MCS, and experimental evidence does not support any one particular immunologic mechanism over another, or for that matter immunologic mechanisms over non-immunologic ones.

Because of the complexity of the immune system, no single assay can test the global integrity or adequacy of immune function in a given individual, even in principle. Indeed, within the broad categories of cellular immunity (reactions mediated by lymphocytes and monocyte/macrophages) and humoral immunity (reactions dependent on antibodies) there are multiple independent functions that must be assessed to characterize an individual's immune response. In this chapter we review aspects of the immune system and of immunologic testing that could be pertinent to potential immunologic contributions to the pathogenesis of MCS.

STRUCTURE AND FUNCTION OF THE IMMUNE SYSTEM AND IMMUNOLOGIC TESTING

The immune response results from a tightly orchestrated network of cellular collaborations. In the first of these, foreign substances are detected with great sensitivity and specificity (the *afferent* limb of the immune response). Next, through a wide variety of mechanisms, antibodies or lytic cells are generated that bind to, or otherwise remove, the offending agent, be it virus, bacterium, or other (the *efferent* limb). A complete review of the myriad types of cells and biochemical mediators involved in the immune response is beyond the scope of this chapter, but an excellent recent overview was done by Unanue.[5] Here, we focus on structural and functional aspects of the immune system that are relevant to the interpretation of studies on MCS.

Immune System Structure

Most immunological studies of MCS have focused on lymphocytes, of which 3 types circulate in the peripheral blood. The first type is the B cell, whose progeny (plasma cells) produce antibodies that are vital to host defense against a wide variety of infectious diseases but also can cause clinically significant tissue damage (i.e., an autoimmune reaction). The damage may be diffuse or organ-specific, depending on the specificity of the antibodies concerned and whether antigen-antibody complexes are formed and deposited in tissues.

The second type of circulating lymphocyte is the T cell. T cells are activated by detection of antigen and then produce a variety of regulatory mediators (termed *cytokines*) that in turn control the activation, proliferation, and effector function of all the cells participating in an immune response. For example, certain T cells exert important effects on antibody production and/or on activation of other T cells. These cells generally express the surface protein CD4 and are termed helper, or CD4-positive (CD4+), T cells. Broadly speaking, CD4+ T cells are responsible for initiating the immune response. The other major class of T cells express CD8, rather than CD4, and function as cytotoxic and suppressor cells that kill host cells expressing foreign antigens and also turn off immune responses. These functions, like those of the CD4+ T cells, entail the production and secretion of many cytokines.

The third major type of circulating lymphocyte is the natural killer (NK) cell, so called because of its ability to kill certain target cells in culture immediately upon removal from the donor (in contrast to cytotoxic T cells, which generally require exposure to antigen for several days before killing activity can be detected). The triggering mechanism of NK cells differs from that of T and B lymphocytes, in that NK cells express a common surface receptor that is *inhibited* from killing by generic molecules expressed by normal cells, while T and B lymphocytes express a huge variety of surface receptors that are *activated* by unique molecules not normally expressed by host cells.

Immune System Function

Abnormalities of immune function can be divided into three categories: (1) immune deficiency, or lack of an immune function needed for protection against opportunistic diseases such as infection; (2) immune activation, or excessive function that results in destruction of host tissues, as happens in autoimmune disease; and (3) hypersensitivity, or excessive reaction to small amounts of specific triggering substances found in the environment. *Immediate hypersensitivity* depends on antibody-coated cells that release immune mediators within minutes or even seconds of contact with the antigen recognized by the antibody. Antibodies that mediate immediate hypersensitivity are of the immunoglobulin E (IgE) type. In contrast, *delayed hypersensitivity* depends on recognition of antigen by lymphocytes and macrophages, and requires recruitment of these cells to the site of the antigen. For this reason, delayed hypersensitivity takes 2–3 days to reach a peak reaction.

These three categories, though conceptually distinct, are oversimplifications. For example, immune deficiency can be due to overproduction of mediators that suppress immune function, and it is believed that autoimmunity can be due to a deficiency in suppressor mechanisms. Similarly, cellular activation is not a monolithic, all-or-none concept. In particular, activated T cells (of both CD4$^+$ and CD8$^+$ subsets) express a multitude of cell-surface proteins that are not expressed by non-activated (resting) cells, but these *activation markers* are not all expressed at the same level on activated T cells (and in some cases are expressed, albeit at lower levels, on resting T cells), as discussed later in this chapter.

Many immune-mediated mechanisms of disease are now known. For example, depletion of CD4$^+$ T-helper cells correlates very strongly with the development of immune deficiency (AIDS) in infection with human immunodeficiency virus, type 1 (HIV-1).[6] Immune activation also is an important feature of HIV-1 infection, and is present in many other diseases. Profound activation of CD8$^+$ T cells occurs in many acute viral infections, and high production of cytokines by these cells contributes to the "malaise" and other symptoms associated with these infections. For example, numbers of activated CD8$^+$ T cells in the peripheral blood may rise to very high levels in infectious mononucleosis, and account for the atypical lymphocytosis that is the hallmark of this disease.[7,8] An increase in activated CD8$^+$ T cells has also been demonstrated in chronic fatigue syndrome.[9] It has long been postulated that imbalances of CD4$^+$ and CD8$^+$ T cells, in number and/or function, could lead to loss of normal regulation of the immune response, but this has been difficult to demonstrate convincingly. Among the diseases where loss of suppressor cells has been claimed to contribute to pathogenesis are putative autoimmune diseases, such as multiple sclerosis[10] and systemic lupus erythematosus.[11] However, whether suppressor cell abnormalities are primary to these disease processes is not known.

Immunophenotyping: An Example of Immune System Testing and Quality Control

In testing for immune abnormalities, it is possible to measure both structure—the extent to which the necessary components of the immune response in question

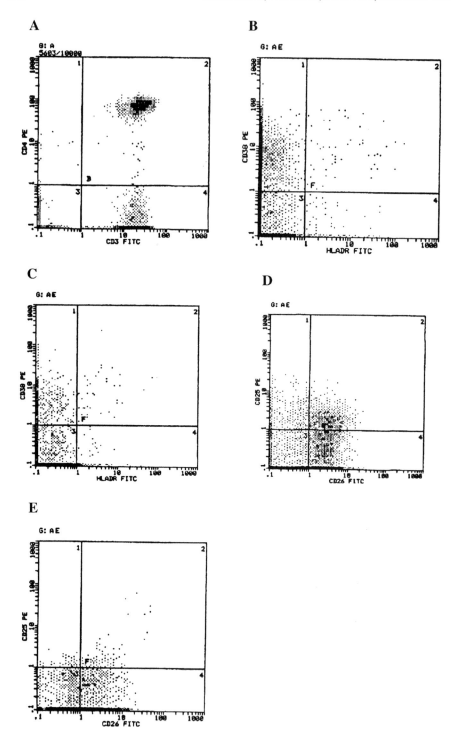

are present—and function—whether they are working as they should. Function and structure are to some extent complementary, and quantitative and qualitative assessment of both are needed. It is also preferable to have a detailed understanding of immune mechanisms in order to select the appropriate test or panel of tests to determine whether an immune abnormality is contributing to a patient's problem. This raises three difficult issues. First, are the specific tests pertinent to the clinical situation in question? Second, are *in vitro* functional tests pertinent to the *in vivo* situation? An abnormal result on a laboratory test, even if the test has been validly performed, as discussed below, does not necessarily indicate an abnormality of immune function *in vivo*. Third, does quantifying structural components of the immune system, which is generally relatively easy and inexpensive, adequately predict immune function, which is generally more complex and expensive to test?

The complexity of these analyses is aptly demonstrated in the case of quantitative measurement of immune cell surface markers, one of the methods most commonly used in previous studies of MCS. It is now possible to measure a large number of these markers with precision and sensitivity using flow cytometry, which provides detailed data on large numbers of individual cells. A detailed description of flow cytometry is beyond the scope of this review, and can be found elsewhere.[12] In brief, cells labeled with fluorescent antibodies are passed through a laser beam at high speeds and the resulting scattering of laser light and emission of laser-excited fluorescence are detected by photomultiplier tubes attached to high speed computers. Flow cytometers are capable of analyzing, and providing quantitative measurements of fluorescence on, thousands of cells per second (Fig. 1). As shown in *A* for CD4+ T cells, the major T cell subsets are characterized by a large difference in the amount of fluorescence between the stained and the unstained cells. This is due to the fact that the surface markers that define these subsets are expressed at a high level, if they are expressed at all. As a result, measurement of these lymphocyte subsets is relatively easy

FIGURE 1 (Opposite Page). Histograms of flow cytometric analyses of T cell phenotypes. In each histogram, two different fluorescence measurements on individual lymphocytes are represented by each dot. The axes depict fluorescence intensity obtained from staining of cells with a monoclonal antibody conjugated to fluorescein isothiocyanate (FITC, *horizontal axis*) and phycoerythrin (PE, *vertical axis*) . The fluorescence intensity is directly related to the amount of antibody bound to each lymphocyte, which in turn is proportional to the level of expression of the surface marker recognized by the monoclonal antibody. For each axis, the background level of staining (derived by staining with isotype control antibodies) is defined by the solid line. For the combination of two antibodies, four possible staining phenotypes are possible and are represented by the numbered quadrants 1–4 defined by the solid lines. Cells that did not stain with either antibody (i.e., cells that have only background fluorescence) would be depicted in quadrant 3.

A, The horizontal axis depicts fluorescence due to expression of CD3 (a marker of T cells), and the vertical axis fluorescence due to CD4 expression. Double-positive cells (quadrant 2) therefore are CD4+ T cells. Note the clear separation of stained cells (quadrants 2 and 4) from unstained cells (quadrant 3). **B–E,** Fluorescence due to expression of the activation markers indicated (CD25, CD26, CD38, and HLA-DR). Note that expression of these markers is not clearly separate from background fluorescence (quadrant 3). **B and C,** Data derived from lymphocytes expressing CD4 in a three-color fluorescence analysis (CD4 data not shown). Dots represent activation marker expression by helper T lymphocytes. **D and E,** Data derived from lymphocytes expressing CD8 in a three-color fluorescence analysis (CD8 data not shown). Dots represent activation marker expression by suppressor-cytotoxic T lymphocytes. Note the differing frequencies and staining intensities of the 4 activation markers, both among themselves and on CD4+ vs. CD8+ T cells.

and forgiving of technical inaccuracy. In particular, these large differences in fluorescence make it possible for an observer using a fluorescence microscope to discriminate stained (fluorescent) from unstained (non-fluorescent) cells. However, just the opposite is true for many of the activation markers, where expression of the pertinent proteins is low, many if not most of the stained cells are only weakly fluorescent, and the intensity of fluorescence appears as a continuum between the unstained and stained cells (see *B–D* for illustrations for some of the activation markers referred to later in the chapter).

Two important points follow from these observations. First, careful attention must be paid to determining the boundary between negative and positive fluorescence, i.e., the level of fluorescence which the cells exhibit in the absence of the specific antibody. This is done with staining controls that use antibodies chemically similar to the antibodies specific for the activation markers, but known not to bind to any markers expressed by the cells being analyzed (i.e., isotype controls). Second, since staining is represented by a continuum of fluorescence, it is difficult, if not impossible, for the observer using a microscope to discriminate positive from negative cells accurately and reliably. Just such a difficulty may have been experienced in at least one of the studies of MCS discussed below.[13,14] Finally, because *in vivo* activation markers are expressed on relatively low proportions of lymphocytes, large numbers of cells (more than can be counted manually) often must be analyzed in order to obtain a statistically precise estimate of the proportion of cells that express the marker in question. Based on these considerations, flow cytometry is an essential method for the accurate measurement of activation markers.

Quality Control in Immunologic Testing

Many immunological tests are now standard in hospital, commercial, and research laboratories worldwide. With the increasing prevalence of diseases whose pathogenesis and/or diagnosis involve an immune component, there has been commensurate effort to ensure that important tests, particularly those used to investigate disease mechanisms or experimental treatments, or to monitor the treatment of individual patients, are performed in a standard manner. Organizations such as the College of American Pathologists and the National Institute for Allergy and Infectious Diseases have instituted programs in which well-characterized samples are sent to laboratories for testing. In some cases replicate samples are sent; this is best done blindly, i.e., without identifying the samples as replicates. This approach to quality control allows determination of intra-laboratory reproducibility as well as inter-laboratory comparability.[15] It is now standard for such immunological measurements as helper and suppressor T cell subsets,[16,17] as well as for serum immunoglobulin (antibody) levels and newer measurements such as the quantity of human immunodeficiency virus type 1 RNA in the plasma. However, there has been little quality control for the other markers pertinent to studies of MCS (an exception is reference 18) and none in the setting of MCS.

Quality control in immunological testing depends on reproducibility of results, both within and between laboratories. This has been a major problem in understanding whether immune abnormalities are present in MCS, not to mention whether, if present, they contribute to its pathogenesis. One important aspect of the problem is that for many immunological tests (and other laboratory tests) it is quite possible to obtain an inaccurate measurement with no obvious indication of this inaccuracy. Thus, tests done only in a single laboratory, or which have not been validated with blind analysis of coded specimens, must be interpreted cautiously. For example, early in one study involving flow cytometric analysis of lymphocyte subsets by one of the authors' laboratories (J.B.M.) and three other laboratories, specimens were shared among all four laboratories. Three laboratories detected a low percentage of NK cells (which are identified by antibodies which stain dimly), while one laboratory detected a higher percentage. Investigation of this discrepancy revealed that each of the three flow cytometers that obtained low values was not optimally calibrated (as it happened, a different defect was present in each case) and was underestimating fluorescence, and that the single laboratory which obtained the high value was correct. Thus, quality control is not democratic! These factors weigh heavily in measurement of expression of activation markers on lymphocytes.

The assessment of lymphocyte activation is further complicated by the fact that the different activation markers are not all expressed to the same extent on a given cell (see Figs. 1B–E). In addition, *in vivo* expression of activation markers by cells (i.e., analyzed soon after isolation of the cells) is often much lower than it is on cells which have been pharmacologically activated *in vitro*. Thus, as is so often the case in immune assessment, assessment of cellular activation is not straightforward. In summary, the biologic complexity of assessing immune activation requires stringent attention to quality control.

THEORIES OF AND EVIDENCE FOR IMMUNOLOGIC MECHANISMS IN MCS

The nature of the afferent and efferent functions of the immune system, and the symptoms caused by ongoing immune reactions, make it plausible that altered immune regulation or activation could be an important disease mechanism in MCS (Fig. 2). Early theories of MCS suggested that individuals had classic or modified allergies, involving IgE- and IgG-mediated reactions to a variety of foods, drugs, chemicals, and molds.[2] However, while there are chemicals that provoke IgE-mediated reactions in the occupational setting, to date studies have not shown any consistent evidence that these mechanisms play a significant role in MCS.[19-21] Other possible mechanisms that involve activation of the immune system, such as abnormalities of circulating complement or immune complex formation, have either not been detected, or in some cases not adequately investigated.[21-23]

Most of the recent focus of immunologic investigations has been on lymphocytes and autoantibodies. These theories, which are not necessarily new, have postulated that there is a "dysregulation" of the immune system, rather than simply an inappropriate activation.[22,24] They focus on damage to T lymphocytes, or alteration of the normal balance of T lymphocyte subsets[22,23] which, it is suggested, result in either altered function or changes in cellular populations or mediators.[24] It has also been proposed that immune complexes or a combination of neurologic and immune markers can be used as indicators of exposure to chemicals, without necessarily invoking a specific mechanism.[25,26]

We reviewed the existing clinical immunologic literature on MCS, which consisted primarily of case series. The studies were obtained from reviews of the etiologic hypotheses of MCS[2,3,20,21,23,24,27] and a MEDLINE search of chemical sensitivity and immunology. We included papers in which: (1) the study or case series specifically referred to chemical sensitivity and immunology; (2) primary data were presented; and (3) other potentially confounding diagnoses (e.g., sick building syndrome or hypersensitivity pneumonitis), if not adequately excluded, at least did not appear to be the primary focus of the investigations. We found seven such papers.

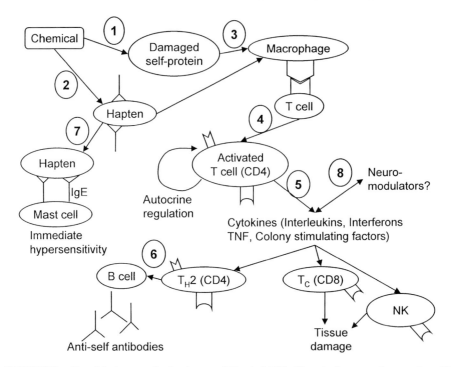

FIGURE 2.   Possible immunologic abnormalities in MCS. Chemicals cause damage to self proteins (1) or react with native chemicals to form hapten-carrier complexes (2). Either mechanism results in recognition and processing by an antigen-processing macrophage (3), which then activates T-cells (4). Through a number of cytokines (interleukins; interferons, especially IFN-γ; tumor necrosis factors [TNF], particularly TNF-α), T-cells, including helper (T_H) and cytotoxic (T_C) and natural killer (NK) cells are activated (5). In some cases B-cells are activated to and differentiate into plasma cells which elaborate antibodies that may attack self-proteins (6). Although considerable time has been spent looking for evidence that MCS involves immediate hypersensitivity through an IgE-mediated pathway (7), thus far there is no evidence of such a reaction. Another hypothesis is that cytokines influence neuropeptides such as substance P (8).

In a case series, Rea et al.[28] examined 12 patients and tested them for IgG, IgE, IgA, IgM, C3 and C4, α-1 anti-trypsin, C-reactive protein, total serum hemolytic complement, and white blood cell counts with differentials. This was a descriptive paper, in which patients served as their own controls. The authors used longitudinal changes in some of the immunologic markers to conclude that a role for complement and IgG was possible.

Heuser et al.[29] studied 135 patients with "sensitivity to small amounts of chemicals" drawn from the investigators' clinical practice, with 160 healthy controls. They measured cell surface markers, specific antibodies, and a variety of physiologic parameters. They described in some detail the quality control techniques used in the laboratory, such as specificity and cross-inhibition of the antibodies used to measure specific antibodies against conjugates of formaldehyde, toluene diisocyanate, phthalic anhydride, and benzene. The abnormality observed most frequently in the chemically sensitive group was higher absolute counts and percentages of lymphocytes expressing the lymphocyte cell surface protein Ta1 (now known as CD26, and discussed below) in cases than in controls. They noted that IgE was not elevated, but found that specific antibodies to chemicals were elevated in patients. Further, in a few patients some of the markers changed over time when putative chemical exposures (not measured directly) were altered. The authors concluded that patients diagnosed with chemical sensitivity can be followed and assessed on the basis of changes in Ta1[+] cells and circulating chemical antibody levels.

Terr[30] reviewed 50 of his patients who had been referred for independent medical evaluations after they had been diagnosed by other physicians with "environmental illness." Of these, 11 cases might not have met a definition of MCS, since symptoms were isolated to a single organ system and could, in the opinion of the author, be attributed to another diagnosis such as bronchial asthma, atopic dermatitis, or temperomandibular joint dislocation with malocclusion (among others). All 50 patients were included in the analysis of immunological markers, based on testing done by the primary care physicians (not the author). No significant differences in immunologic markers were observed, although the inclusion of patients with diverse diagnoses potentially limits the conclusions that can be drawn regarding chemical sensitivity.

McGovern et al.[31] compared six chemically sensitive patients with "multisystemic clinical syndromes" characterized by "extreme hypersensitivity reactions to many food and inhalant allergens," as well as positive intradermal skin whealing when challenged by most of the 40 common allergen extracts, with six subjects who had no symptoms of allergy. Both groups were challenged with either foods to which they (the cases) were sensitive or chemicals that had provoked their symptoms. This study is noteworthy because subjects were provocatively challenged and their acute response to the challenge (levels of serotonin, histamine, total hemolytic complement, epinephrine, dopamine, and prostaglandin $F_{2\alpha}$) were recorded. The authors concluded, based on the provocative challenges with what were supposed to be patient-specific materials, that chemically sensitive individuals demonstrated type 1 (immediate hypersensitivity) and/or type 3 (deposition of antigen-antibody complexes) immune responses, compared with no responses by controls. However, again it may be difficult to make definitive conclusions because of the diversity of diagnoses among the cases.

Kipen et al.[32] reported preliminary data on 11 patients diagnosed with MCS, compared with 11 healthy male farmers and 7 patients with chronic fatigue syndrome. The investigators looked at cell mediated immunity, cell counts, complement, immunoglobulins, and cell surface activation markers. Although these were preliminary results, the authors observed an increase among MCS patients of elevated CD4/CD8 ratios, due to low percentages of CD8[+] T-cells.

Simon et al.[13] studied 41 patients with chemical sensitivity (recruited from a physician's clinical practice) and 34 controls with chronic musculoskeletal disorders which were presumed to be non-immunologic. The investigators looked at autoantibodies and changes in lymphocyte populations, as well as selected cytokines. Their findings regarding immunologic markers—that there were few substantial differences between cases and controls—have been questioned due to concerns about the sensitivity and reliability of the analytical methods used.[14]

Finally, Ziem and McTamney[33] reported an uncontrolled study of 68 patients with MCS seen in a clinical practice. This case series compared a large number of immunologic tests done at different laboratories over time. Some immunologic abnormalities were described compared to laboratory normal values, notably high levels of total Ta1[+] (CD26[+]) lymphocytes and selected autoantibodies. As with the other case series, quality control measures were not described, and the authors did not describe their criteria for inclusion of cases.

Table 1 summarizes our evaluation of these studies with respect to some conventional clinical and epidemiologic criteria. First, was an *a priori* case definition used to select cases, or were cases defined after the fact (*Case Definition*)? Only three of the seven studies described a case definition that was prospectively applied to the subjects; most relied on a clinical diagnosis made by a treating physician.

Second, who established the diagnosis (*Diagnosis*)? In two of the studies, diagnoses were made by referring physicians rather than by either the investigator or an independent clinician using a standardized case definition. Studies in which diagnoses were not independently verified left open the possibility of misdiagnosis or inconsistent application of a case definition.

We have already discussed some of the issues involved in using standard reference values for comparison. The majority (4/7) of the investigations used the testing immunology laboratory's population reference values (no controls), while the remainder (3/7) used another reference group selected by the investigators (controls). Some studies used healthy controls, while others used control groups with non-immunologic health problems or other immune conditions. While each of these controls has advantages and disadvantages, we considered either preferable to the use of the diagnostic laboratory's definition of "Normal."

Most of the studies (5/7) had a standardized battery of tests (*Test Selection*) that were applied to all of the subjects. In two of the case series, the studies were individually selected for clinical purposes, making it more difficult to compare all of the subjects in the study.

In addition to whether the studies had internal controls, we also looked at whether the investigators relied primarily on the laboratory's definition of "normal" ranges for lab values (*Normal Range*). Even some studies with internal controls in some cases (2/7) relied primarily on the lab, rather than constructing internal norms.

One of the primary emphases of this chapter has been the importance of quality control (*Quality Control*). Only one of seven papers described the quality control program in sufficient detail to inspire confidence in the procedures used. This was a major shortcoming of the studies reviewed. A similar limitation was the lack of description of the statistical analysis applied to the laboratories' immunological data (*Analysis*). Only one study described the methods of analysis sufficiently to allow evaluation of the data.

In addition to the above studies on MCS, Thrasher and Broughton published data on immune activation in workers in buildings with poor air quality and workers exposed to organic chemicals. Although these studies do not deal with MCS directly and thus are excluded from the table, they are often cited in connection with MCS because they claim to show that an antibody response can arise from exposure to low concentrations of common organic chemicals. Specifically, these authors reported the presence of IgG antibodies to formaldehyde- and toluene diisocyanate-albumin conjugates.[15,19] There were, however, no control subjects in the study, so it is difficult to interpret the results. Further, since the patients in these studies were not diagnosed with MCS or selected on the basis of MCS criteria, it is difficult to extrapolate the results to MCS. Finally, these studies involved exposures at higher concentrations than those typically seen in MCS, and the health effects seen were more typical of immunologic responses such as hypersensitivity pneumonitis.

Taken as a whole, this review demonstrates that the current literature on immunological mechanisms and abnormalities in MCS is still at a very early stage. All

TABLE 1. Selected Previous Studies of Immunologic Abnormalities in MCS Patients

Study	Patients	Findings	A priori Case Definition	Source of Diagnosis	Controls	Test Selection	Normal Range	Quality Control	Analytic Method
					Attributes				
Rea et al.[28]	Case series of 12 patients	Decreased T-cell percentages	N	ND	N	F	—	ND	N
McGovern et al.[31]	6 patients with 6 healthy controls, challenged with petrochemical inhalants	Abnormal baseline T- and B-cell levels; both IgE and IgG implicated in challenge response	Y	ND	Y	F	Lab	ND	N
Terr[30]	50 patients referred for "environmentally induced illness"; 43/50 referred for Workers' Compensation claim	No consistent pattern of abnormalities in numbers, percentages of T, B, or null cells, T-cell subsets, complement, antinuclear antibody; 4 patients with elevated IgA	N	Ref MD	N	V	Lab	ND	ND
Kipen et al.[32]	11 patients referred for MCS, meeting criteria and physician-diagnosed; controls are 11 male farmers with hypertension only, and 7 patients with CSF	5/11 MCS patients had abnormally high CD4/CD8 ratios, compared with 2 of the healthy controls and 1 of the CFS controls	Y	Inv	Y	F	Lab	ND	ND
Heuser et al.[29]	135 patients with physician-diagnosed MCS from a clinic population, 160 healthy controls	Increased percentage of Ta1 (CD26)+ lymphocytes, variable CD4/CD8 ratios, and longitudinal changes in antibodies to chemical-protein conjugates	N	Inv	N	F	Inv	ND	N
Simon et al.[13]	41 patients with physician-diagnosed MCS, 34 controls with musculoskeletal injuries	No difference in autoantibodies; lymphocyte count; percentages of T or B cells, IL2 receptor (CD25)+ cells, or Ta1 (CD26)+ cells; or generation of IL-1 *in vitro*; CD4+ lymphocyte percentage greater in cases	Y	Ref MD	Y	F	Inv	Y	Y
Ziem and McTamney[33]	68 patients from clinical practice, no controls	Increased total Ta1 (CD26)+ (95%); anti-myelin and antismooth muscle autoantibodies in 43% and 53%, respectively	ND	Inv	N	V	Lab	ND	N

ND = Not described, V = Variable, Inv = Done by investigators, Ref MD = Done by referring physician, Y = yes, N = No, F = Fixed set of variables, Lab = Defined by laboratory.

of the available studies have limitations that make it difficult to reach any conclusions regarding the role of immunology in MCS, such as a lack of a consistent case definition, appropriate reference or control groups, and appropriate quality control programs. Some studies also had very small sample sizes. Given the current data, it is not possible to reach firm conclusions about the role of immunological mechanisms (or absence thereof) in the pathogenesis and diagnosis of MCS.

VALIDATION AND EVALUATION OF IMMUNOLOGIC TESTS USED IN MCS

To address some of the issues that have not been resolved by the studies in Table 1, we have recently undertaken a validation study of several of the immunological tests previously used in MCS studies. In particular, we wanted to apply some of the quality control procedures previously described to some of the markers that have been claimed to support a diagnosis of MCS. The study had two phases. The first involved a test of the reproducibility of selected immunological parameters commonly tested in MCS, and the second compared selected immunological parameters in patients with and without a physician-confirmed diagnosis of MCS.

In the first phase, the laboratories that chose to participate have a record of being involved either in testing of patients suspected to have MCS—Immunosciences and Specialty Laboratories, both in Los Angeles, CA—or in quality control efforts in immunological testing—Johns Hopkins University (JHU), University of Washington, and Rutgers University, New Jersey; and autoantibody laboratories at JHU and Scripps Research Institute, La Jolla, CA. The study involved duplicate blinded specimens sent to each laboratory, drawn from donors at JHU. Blood was drawn from volunteers who either had no known disease, were known to have an immunological disease, or had MCS according to a physician or by self-report. Since the goal of the study was to evaluate "real-world" laboratory performance, not to optimize it, we did not collect detailed information about laboratory methods or donor diagnoses. Blood was immediately divided into aliquots that were either sent to the local laboratories for analysis the same day or shipped to participating laboratories by overnight mail for analysis the next day. Each laboratory received two masked replicate samples from each donor. Samples from multiple patients were sent together, so that no assumption could be made as to how samples were paired. Since the freshly analyzed and overnight-shipped samples yielded similar results at the local laboratory, we concentrate here on the results obtained on the shipped samples.

The immunological tests performed in this study were chosen on the basis of previous reports of immune abnormalities in MCS, as discussed above. These included the major T cell subsets (CD4$^+$ and CD8$^+$) and some activation markers previously studied in MCS: CD25, the α chain of the interleukin-2 receptor; CD26 (formerly known as Ta1), the cell surface enzyme dipeptidyl peptidase IV; and HLA-DR, the human class II histocompatibility antigen. Another activation marker included, CD38, has not been studied in MCS but has been extensively studied in HIV-1 infection,[34,35] which as mentioned is characterized by a high level of immune activation,[36–38] and in chronic fatigue syndrome.[9]

An example of measurements of replicate samples illustrating laboratory performance is shown in Figure 3. Conventionally, with acceptable laboratory performance most replicate measurements of T cell subsets would be expected to be within 2% of each other. For the example shown, it can be seen that this was indeed true in most cases.

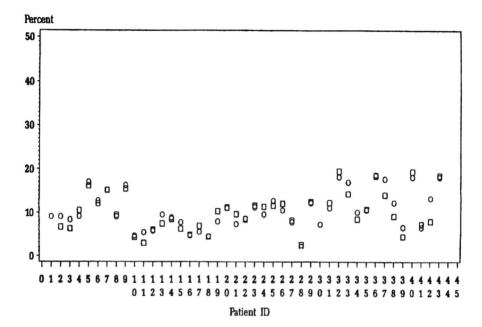

FIGURE 3. Replicate values for the measurement of the proportion of lymphocytes expressing both CD25 and CD4, using data from one laboratory which received blinded replicate specimens as described in the text. The vertical axis indicates the measured percentage of lymphocytes expressing both CD25 and CD4, and the horizontal axis indicates the specimen number. The results obtained in the analyses of the two replicate samples are depicted by a circle and a square for each replicate analyzed. Agreement is generally very close, but note disparate replicates for specimens 37 and 42.

Representative data comparing laboratories for selected T cell subsets are shown in Figure 4. For the CD4+ T cell subset (A), previously illustrated as a relatively simple measurement technically, agreement was very close across all laboratories. However, for the CD25+ subset of T cells (B), the data were much more variable, consistent with the greater difficulty of this measurement as discussed above. In fact, significant inter-laboratory variation was found for most of the activation markers, as well as the major T cell subsets, although the latter differences were much smaller. These findings will be described in detail elsewhere (manuscript in preparation).

Another way of looking at reproducibility data is to examine the bias of a particular laboratory in a given measurement across multiple patients. This is done by calculating the difference between the measurement in that laboratory and the mean of the other laboratories which analyzed an aliquot of the same specimen (Fig. 5). The value of this type of analysis, combined with other analyses described above, is to prevent a "rush to judgment" by identifying apparent trends in cell markers that may actually be due to consistent differences between laboratories.

After analyzing results from the phase one study, it was possible to study whether any of the tests validated in phase one would be useful in distinguishing patients with and without MCS (phase two). For this study, we used a case definition that included symptoms in three or more organ systems with exposure; symptoms

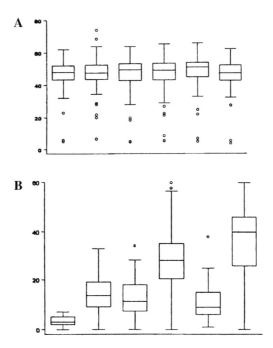

FIGURE 4. Box plot displays of measurements of A) CD4+ lymphocytes and B) CD25 expression on T cells in the specimens shared among the participating laboratories. The vertical axis indicates the percentage of lymphocytes that express CD4 in A) and both CD25 and CD3 in B). The horizontal axis indicates the 6 laboratories. Boxes indicate the 25th, 50th, and 75th percentiles of the distributions, and arms indicate the ranges of the values, except for outliers which are indicated by circles. Note the excellent agreement in A) and the wide range of values in B).

were chronic and occurred at or below previously tolerated levels of exposure. Key in this phase were two considerations: (1) using tests and laboratories that were validated; and (2) rigorously screening patient groups to minimize patient misclassification. The first aspect has been discussed above; the second is discussed in detail in the full report of the study (in preparation). In brief, candidates for the MCS group underwent both a pre-screening aimed at excluding people with MCS who had potentially confounding conditions, and, if not excluded, a clinical and laboratory examination for other diseases that could affect the immunologic tests performed. Approximately one-third of the patients who passed the initial screening for MCS were not enrolled in the study following the clinical and laboratory evaluation, either because of the presence of other potentially confounding conditions or because they did not meet our case definition of MCS. Twenty-three people were enrolled in the MCS group. In addition, the control group was screened to rule out the presence of MCS, and twenty-one people were enrolled.

Even with the laboratory validation procedures that have been explained above, we felt it necessary to include two laboratories to perform the T cell subset analyses and two for the antibody analyses of the study populations, to see whether the laboratories would achieve the same findings when the two groups were compared. Indeed, most of the statistically significant differences that were observed between

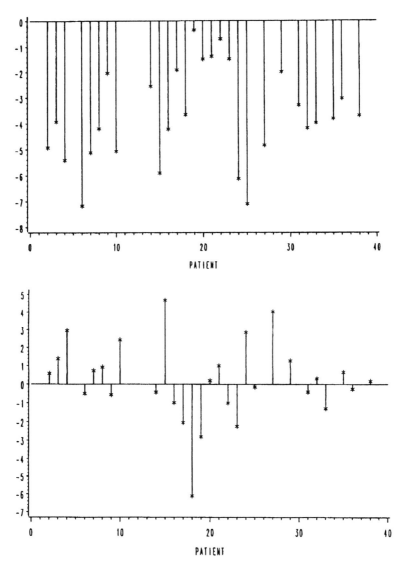

FIGURE 5.   Analyses of laboratory bias. Each figure depicts data from one laboratory. The vertical axis represents the differences, for each specimen, between the percentage of lymphocytes expressing both CD8 and CD38 (i.e., expressing the CD8+CD38+ phenotype) measured by the laboratory concerned and the overall mean of the measurements by all five laboratories. The horizontal axis represents the donor number.

the MCS group and the healthy group were observed in one laboratory but not both. This suggests that further work is needed to define the utility of immunological testing, at least with respect to the tests performed in this study. Considered as a whole and compared to the healthy controls, the MCS group did not differ in most immunological measurements. The only exception thus far was the finding that CD4+ lymphocyte percentages were higher, and CD8+ percentages lower, in the group with

MCS compared to the group with no disease. These findings are similar to those obtained by Kipen et al.[32] Analysis of data from the study is still ongoing, and a full description of this study will be published elsewhere.

CONTROVERSIES

Is MCS a disorder of immune regulation? There are both theoretical grounds and some experimental evidence to support the notion that some chemicals can alter immune function, both by activating it and, in some cases, by suppressing it. Theoretically, there are compounds that can affect the immune system, either by eliciting specific immune responses, or by global effects on cell lineages. The nature of the reported symptoms in MCS is consistent with a systemic response to some external agent. Particularly if other systems are included in the discussion, it is not unreasonable to think that neuro-immune interactions could be affected by a toxin, resulting in symptoms of the type reported. Some limited experimental evidence also supports such a mechanism. For example, several studies (reviewed here in Table 1) have identified a relative increase in the proportion of $CD26^+$ ($Ta1^+$) cells in MCS cases.

However, there are several problems with this notion, both theoretical and based on experimental evidence. These have been thoroughly discussed in several reviews on the subject.[3,22,27] First, the hallmark of the immune system is its specificity. The notion that a diverse array of chemically dissimilar compounds would elicit a common subtle pathway of immune dysregulation is not supported by any current clinical findings, or any known immunological mechanism. Although it is quite possible to suppress or damage the immune response through application of physical and biological agents, these effects are generally not subtle. Theories that rely on complex interactions between the immune system and other systems, for example the neurological or endocrine systems, have become so complex that they are both difficult to explain mechanistically and, at least so far, impossible to test experimentally.

The studies that have been done up to now have sufficient methodological limitations (e.g., lack of appropriate controls, absence of consistent case definitions, problems with the immunologic tests performed, limited sample size) that it is difficult if not impossible to validate any etiologic hypothesis based on the immunologic data. For example, in some previous studies of MCS, patients with airways disease, including RADS, rhinitis, or asthma, may have been included in the study population, while in other studies these individuals would have been excluded for not meeting the study case definition. This inconsistency has important implications for the clinical evaluation and management of patients who may present with concerns about MCS, as well as for the validity of previous clinical studies of immunologic markers in MCS.

In the opinion of the authors, there is no single etiologic hypothesis of MCS that would suggest a narrow evaluation of selected immunologic parameters. As demonstrated by the review of existing literature, no consistent pattern of immunologic abnormalities has been shown to date, and further testing of clinic populations with batteries of immunologic assays seems likely to offer little improvement over the current state of knowledge. For example, elevated $CD4^+/CD8^+$ T cell ratios, which were observed in some of the reviewed studies, were of small magnitude; thus, even if elevated ratios were consistently found in groups of people with MCS, this measurement would still not be clinically useful for an individual patient in view of its wide normal range. Furthermore, most expert panels and consensus statements have either discounted an immunologic basis for MCS or recommended symptom-based approaches to immunologic testing, rather than specific recommended test batteries.[39–42] However, there is a (general) need to improve the utility of diagnostic immunologic testing, and to define areas where evaluation of selected, biologically relevant immunologic markers can be evaluated in well defined clinical or general populations. There are also opportunities to improve the clinical utility of immunologic tests, by subjecting laboratories to the same kind of rigorous quality control and validation that has been accomplished for tests that are essential for the diagnosis and management of other diseases.

Finally, two areas where further research might be helpful are: (1) evaluation of immunological markers in patients during controlled challenges with specific chemicals; and (2) population-based evaluation of immunological markers, using appropriate quality control measures. Findings from these types of research could then be applied to prospective, longitudinal evaluations of MCS.

CONCLUSION

Although there has been much speculation about the possible role of the immune system in the etiology of MCS, there remains little or no firm evidence to support such a role. Previous studies have been limited in three key respects: (1) the absence of testable hypotheses and selection of tests based on an hypothesis; (2) difficulties in selection of appropriate and well-defined cases and controls; and (3) limitations in the appropriate validation and quality control of immunologic tests used. While immunological testing has an important role in the diagnosis and management of specific immune disorders, the use of immunological tests as screening tools, to identify or diagnose MCS, is unwarranted due to the limitations noted above. Patients should be informed that subtle differences in individual immunological parameters, especially if observed in only one laboratory, are common and do not necessarily indicate the presence of a systemic disorder, unless there are additional clinical correlates and the results are verified. To the extent that further exploratory research is justified in this area, it should involve well-validated measures with appropriate quality control, well-defined clinical groups, and possibly specific chemical challenges.

ACKNOWLEDGEMENTS

We thank the study participants and the directors at the participating laboratories. We thank Grace Ziem, MD, MPH, Michelle Petri, MD, Paul Ladenson, MD, and Marge Evert, RN for help with patient recruitment; Karen Eckert-Kohl, Nicole Carpinetti, and Ellen Taylor for technical assistance; Joshua Shinoff for scheduling of study participants; Stacey Meyerer and Cynthia King for data entry; Joshua Shinoff and Dongguang Li for data management and statistical analysis; Rhonda Austin, Maggie Shaw, Amy Alfriend, Maureen Thompson and the staff at the Johns Hopkins Center for Occupational and Environmental Health for subject evaluation; and Drs. Brian Schwartz and Virginia Weaver for clinical evaluations. The study was supported by a grant from the Washington State Department of Labor and Industry.

REFERENCES

1. Cullen MR: The worker with multiple chemical sensitivities: An overview. Occup Med 2:655–661, 1987.
2. Levin AS, Byers VS: Environmental illness: A disorder of immune regulation. Occup Med 2:669–681, 1987.
3. Sparks PJ, Daniell W, Black D, et al: Multiple chemical sensitivity syndrome: A clinical perspective. J Occup Env Med 36:718–730, 1994.
4. Miller CS: Toxicant-induced loss of tolerance—an emergent theory of disease? Environ Health Perspec 105S2:445–453, 1997.

5. Unanue ER: Overview of the immune system. In Frank MM, Austen KF, Claman HN, et al (eds): Samter's Immunologic Diseases. 5th ed., Vol 1. Boston, Little, Brown and Company, 1995, pp 3–16.
6. Fauci AS: Immunopathogenic mechanisms in HIV-1 infection. Ann Intern Med 114:678–693, 1991.
7. Callan MFC, Steven N, Krausa P, et al: Large clonal expansions of CD8+ T cells in acute infectious mononucleosis. Nature Medicine 2:906–911, 1996.
8. Carney WP, Rubin RH, Hoffman RA, et al: Analysis of T lymphocytes subsets in cytomegalovirus mononucleosis. J Immunol 126:2114–2116, 1981.
9. Landay A, Jessop C, Lennette ET, et al: Chronic fatigue syndrome: Clinical condition associated with immune activation. Lancet 338:707–712, 1991.
10. Morimoto CM, et al.: Selective loss of the suppressor-inducer T-cell subset in progressive multiple sclerosis. Analysis with anti-2H4 monoclonal antibody. N Engl J Med 316:67, 1987.
11. Horwitz DA, Stohl W: T lymphocytes, cytokines, and immune regulation in systemic lupus erythematosus. In Wallace DJ, Hahn BH (eds): Dubois' Lupus Erythematosus, 4th ed. Philadelphia, Lea & Febiger, 1993, pp 83–96.
12. Parks DR, Herzenberg LA: Flow cytometry and fluorescence-activated cell sorting: theory, experimental optimization, and applications in lymphoid cell biology. Methods Enzymology 108:197–241, 1989.
13. Simon GE, Daniell W, Stockbridge H, et al: Immunologic, psychological, and neuropsychological factors in multiple chemical sensitivity: a controlled study. Ann Intern Med 119:97–103, 1993.
14. Margolick JB, Vogt RF: Controversy over multiple chemical sensitivities (letter). Ann Intern Med 220:249–249, 1994.
15. Koepke JA, Landay AL: Precision and accuracy of absolute lymphocyte counts. Clin Immunol Immunopathol 52:19–27, 1989.
16. Kagan J, Gelman R, Waxdal M, et al: Quality Assessment Program. Annals of NY Acad of Sci 677:50, 1993.
17. Paxton H, Kidd P, Landay A, et al: Results of the flow cytometry ACTG quality control program: Analysis and findings. Clin Immunol Immunopathol 52:68–84, 1989.
18. Landay AL, Brambilla D, Pitts J, et al: Interlaboratory variability of CD8 subset measurements by flow cytometry and its applications to multicenter clinical trials. Clin Diagnostic Lab Immunol 2:462–468, 1995.
19. Broughton A, Thrasher JD, Gard Z: Immunological evaluation of our arc welders exposed to fumes from ignited polyurethane (isocyanate) foam: Antibodies and immune profiles. Am J Indust Med 13:463–472, 1988.
20. Bernstein DI: Multiple chemical sensitivity: State of the art symposium: The role of chemical allergens. Reg Toxicol Pharmacol 24:S28–S31, 1996.
21. Albright JF, Goldstein RA: Is there evidence of an immunologic basis for multiple chemical sensitivity? Toxicol Indust Health 8:215–219, 1992.
22. Salvaggio JE: Understanding clinical immunological testing in alleged chemically induced environmental illnesses. Regul Toxicol Pharmacol 24:S16–S27, 1996.
23. Terr AI: Multiple chemical sensitivities: immunologic critique of clinical ecology theories and practice. Occup Med 2:683–695, 1987.
24. Meggs WJ: Immunological mechanisms of disease and the multiple chemical sensitivity syndrome. In Multiple Chemical Sensitivities: Addendum to biologic markers in immunotoxicology. National Research Council, Washington, DC, National Academy Press, 1992, pp 155–168.
25. Dietert RR, Hedge A: Chemical sensitivity and the immune system: A paradigm to approach potential immune involvement. NeuroToxicol 19:253–257, 1998.
26. Kreutzer R, Neutra RR, Lashuay N: Use of laboratory tests for immune biomarkers in environmental health studies concerned with exposure to indoor air pollutants. Environ Health Perspec 95:85–9112, 1991.
27. Graveling RA, Pilkington A, George PK, et al: A review of multiple chemical sensitivity. Occupat Environ Med 56:73–85, 1999.
28. Rea WJ, Bell IR, Suits CW, et al: Food and chemical susceptibility after environmental chemical overexposure: Case histories. Ann.Allergy 41:101–110, 1978.
29. Heuser G, Wojdani A, Heuser S: Diagnostic markers of multiple chemical sensitivity. In Multiple Chemical Sensitivities: Addendum to Biologic Markers in Immunotoxicology. Washington, DC, National Academy Press, 1992, pp 117–138.
30. Terr AI: Environmental illness: A clinical review of 50 cases. Arch Intern Med 146:145–149, 1986.
31. McGovern JJ Jr, Lazaroni JA, Hicks MF, et al: Food and chemical sensitivity: Clinical and immunologic correlates. Arch Otolaryngol Head Neck Surg 109:292–297, 1983.
32. Kipen H, Fiedler N, Maccia C, et al: Immunologic evaluation of chemically sensitive patients. Toxicol Ind Health 8:125–135, 1992.

33. Ziem G, McTamney J: Profile of patients with chemical injury and sensitivity. Environ Health Perspect 105:417–436, 1997.
34. Liu Z, Hultin LE, Cumberland WG, et al: Elevated relative fluorescence intensity of CD38 antigen expression on CD8+ T cells is a marker of poor prognosis in HIV infection: Results of 6 years of follow-up. Cytometry 26:1–7, 1996.
35. Liu Z, Cumberland WG, Hultin LE, et al: CD8+ T-lymphocyte activation in HIV-1 disease reflects an aspect of pathogenesis distinct from viral burden and immunodeficiency. J Aquir Immune Def Syndr 18:332–340, 1998.
36. Ascher MS, Sheppard HW: AIDS as immune system activation: A model for pathogenesis. Clin Exp Immunol 73:165–170, 1988.
37. Ascher MS, Sheppard HW: AIDS as immune system activation. II. The panergic imnesia hypothesis. J Acquir Immune Defic Syndr 3:177–191, 1990.
38. Fahey JL, Taylor JMG, Detels R, et al: The prognostic value of cellular and serologic markers in infection with human immunodeficiency virus type 1. N Engl J Med 322:166–172, 1990.
39. AAAAI Board of Directors: Position statement: Idiopathic environmental intolerance. Allerg Clin Immunol 103:36–40, 1999.
40. American College of Physicians: Position paper: Clinical ecology. Ann Intern Med 111:168–178, 1989.
41. Council on Scientific Affairs AMA: Clinical ecology. JAMA 268:1634–1635, 1992.
42. McLellan RK, Becker CE, Borak JB, et al: Multiple chemical sensitivities: Idiopathic environmental intolerance. J Occup Environ Med 41:940–942, 1999.

INDEX

Entries in **boldface type** indicate complete chapters.

Abused building syndrome. *See* Sick building syndrome
Acetone exposure, odor perception and irritation responses to, 546–547, 550–551
Acquired immunodeficiency syndrome (AIDS)
  CD4⁺ T cell deficiency associated with, 649
  as neuropsychological deficit cause, 620
Activities of daily living (ADLs) impairments, in IEI patients, 498, 622, 629
Advocacy and support groups, for IEI patients, 551, 563, 564, 629, 631–632, 633, 634
Affective disorders, in IEI patients, 622–624
Affective inhibition, in IEI patients, 561
Affectivity, negative
  effect on odor sensitivity, 547–549, 552
  as IEI risk factor, relationship to behavioral conditioning, 523
Agoraphobia, toxic, 560
Air Force personnel, Gulf War syndrome in, 588, 591
Air pollutants, indoor. *See also* Sick building syndrome
  exposure limits for, 575, 576–577
  immunologic response to, 656
Airway irritation, chemical exposure-related, effect of attention level on, 549–550
Alcohol abuse/alcoholism
  in family members of IEI patients, 565
  lack of association with IEI, 567
Aldehydes, as sick building syndrome cause, 575, 581
Alternative treatment, of IEI, 563, 608
Alzheimer's disease
  brain imaging-assisted diagnosis of, 612
  as neuropsychological deficit cause, 620
American Academy of Allergy and Immunology, 507
American Academy of Neurology, 612
American College of Occupational and Environmental Medicine, 507
American College of Physicians, 507
American Council on Science and Health, 507–508
American Medical Association, Council of Scientific Affairs, 507, 557, 582
American Society for Heating, Refrigerating, and Air-Conditioning Engineers, 579, 580
Anger, of IEI patients, 629
Antibody response, to chemical exposure, 655, 656
Antidepressants, as IEI therapy, 608, 639, 640

Antisocial personality disorder
  antipsychotic drug therapy for, 632
  in family of IEI patients, 565
  in IEI patients, 634
  lack of association with IEI, 567, 568
Anxiety/anxiety disorders
  anticipatory, as panic attack cause, 504
  IEI-associated, 504, 558, 559–560, 561, 568, 623, 627, 628, 634
    brain imaging studies of, 502
    as conditioned response, 523
    desensitization treatment for, 536
    pharmacological treatment for, 607–608
    treatment model for, 638–639
  as neuropsychological deficit cause, 620
  effect on olfactory sensitivity, 503, 504
  personality disorder-related, 632
Asthma
  in Gulf War veterans, 593
  stereotypic stress response in, 525
Asthma attacks, psychogenic, 506
Atopy, 574, 578, 582
Attention deficits, in IEI patients, 629
  depression-/anxiety-related, 502
  quantitative electroencephalographic therapy for, 636
Attention level, effect on chemosensory response, 545, 549–550
Autointoxication, 630
Autonomic reactivity, of IEI patients, 540, 542
Avoidance behavior, of IEI patients, 565
  to aversive chemicals, 521
    case report of, 563, 564
    deleterious effects of, 608
  for primary gain, 632
  treatment of, 560, 637
Avoidant personality disorder, in IEI patients, 562
Axis I disorders, in IEI patients, 559, 563
Axis II disorders, in IEI patients, 559

B cells, 648
Behavioral conditioning, **519–528**. *See also* Pavlovian conditioning
  in IEI, 499, 503–504, 521–527
    conditioned immunomodulation, 521–522, 527
    of conditioned odor and taste aversions, 521, 522–524, 527
    implication for treatment, 525–527
    individual differences in, 525, 527
    of pharmacologic sensitization, 524, 527
    odor-guided aversive, 522–524
    principles of, 519–521

Behavioral therapy, for IEI, 525–527, 606, 607, 633, 636
  for avoidance behavior, 560, 637
Belief systems, closed, of IEI patients, 634. *See also* Illness belief system, of IEI patients
Bioaerosols, as sick building syndrome cause, 573, 574
Biofeedback, electromagnetic, as IEI therapy, 636
Biological monitoring, of IEI patients, 604
Blood enzyme assays, for porphyria diagnosis, 606
Blood flow, cerebral, in hypocarbia, 504
Blood tests, for exogenous chemicals, 606
Bodily sensations, IEI patients' hypersensitivity to, 562, 622, 633
Borderline personality disorder patients, opposition to psychotropic drug therapy by, 632
Brain, perfusion of, hypocarbia-related decrease in, 504
Brain electrical activity mapping (BEAM), 605
"Brain fog," 504, 629
Brain imaging, in IEI, 502, 605, **611–616**
  with positron emission tomography (PET), 605, 611–612
    contraindication for diagnostic use, 615
  with single-positron emission computed tomography (SPECT), 612, 614
    contraindication for diagnostic use, 615
    inadequate study design of, 613, 614–615
Brain injury, anoxic, as neuropsychological deficits cause, 620
Building-related occupant complaint. *See* Sick building syndrome

California Medical Association, 507
Candidiasis, IEI-associated, 630
Carbon dioxide, exposure limits for, 576
Carbon dioxide (35%) inhalation, as pancogenic stimuli, 529–530, 532, 536
Carbon disulfide, neurotoxicity of, 619
Carbon monoxide
  exposure limits for, 576
  neurotoxicity of, 619
Cardiopulmonary illness, as neuropsychological deficit cause, 620
Case definitions, of IEI, **511–517**
  in clinical cases, 511–515
  in immunologic studies, 656, 657
  in population-based studies, 515–516
Causal relationship, between IEI and chemical exposure, 601–602, 630–631
CD4+ T cells
  CD8+ T cell ratio of, in IEI, 655, 657, 662
  depletion of, 649
  flow cytometric analysis of, 650–652
  as IEI marker, 648, 658, 659, 660
CD8+ T cells, as IEI marker, 655, 658, 661–662
CD25 T cells, as IEI marker, 658, 659, 660
CD26 T cells, as IEI marker, 654–656, 657, 662
CD38 T cells, as IEI marker, 658, 661

Center for Epidemiological Studies-Depression Scale (CES-D), 618
Central nervous system disorders
  IEI-related prevalence of, 498
  infections, as neuropsychological deficits cause, 620
Cerebral allergy. *See* Idiopathic environmental intolerances
Cerebrovascular disease, as neuropsychological deficits cause, 620
Chemical exposure
  causal relationship with IEI, 601–602, 630–631
  confirmation of, 602
  control of, for IEI prevention, 507
  duration and intensity of, 602
  physicians' estimation of, 603
Chemical hypersensitivity syndrome. *See* Idiopathic environmental intolerances (IEI)
Chemical Odor Tolerance Scale, 588–589
Chemical sensitivity
  definition of, 588
  in Gulf War syndrome patients, 566–567, 589, 590, 591, 592
  prevalence of
    in general population, 498, 539, 589
    in Gulf War syndrome patients, 589, 590, 591, 592
  screening instruments for, 588–589
Chemical warfare agents, as Gulf War syndrome cause, 588
Childhood trauma
  as anxiety risk factor, 638
  as IEI risk factor, 565
    implication for psychotherapy, 637–638, 639, 641, 642
  as post-traumatic stress disorder risk factor, 639–640
Chronic fatigue syndrome
  behavior therapy for, 607
  brain imaging studies of, 502, 605, 613–615
  CD8+ T cell activation in, 649
  in Gulf War veterans, 592, 593
  psychotherapy guidelines for, 635
  relationship with IEI, 506, 540, 630
Chronic pain
  behavior therapy for, 607
  psychotherapy for, 641
Civil litigation, by IEI patients, 634
  implication for psychotherapy, 639
Clinical ecologists, 505, 512. *See also* Physicians, environmental
  diagnostic approach of, 512, 514
  IEI case definition of, 513
  need for regulation of, 507
  promotion of IEI diagnoses by, 560
Cocaine, as panic attack cause, 504
Cognitive-behavioral therapy, for IEI, 526, 608, 636–637
Cognitive distortions, 637–638
Cognitive dysfunction
  in Gulf War syndrome patients, 588

Cognitive dysfunction (*cont.*)
  in IEI patients, 502
    relationship to chemical exposure level, 622, 623
  IEI patients' lack of, 621–622, 629
Cognitive factors, in olfactory sensitization, 551–552, 553
Cognitive style, of IEI patients, 631, 633–634
Cognitive therapy, for IEI, 526. *See also* Cognitive-behavioral therapy
Complement, as IEI marker, 657
Compulsive personality disorder. *See also* Obsessive-compulsive disorder
  in IEI patients, 562
Conditioned stimulus-response, in IEI, 623
Conditioning. *See* Behavioral conditioning
Consultations, in diagnostic evaluation of IEI patients, 602, 603
Contagion, epidemic, 631–632
Convergence, 631
Conversion disorders, in IEI patients, 559
  case example of, 564
Corproporphyrin oxidase assay, 606
Criegee radicals, 575, 581
Cults, medical, IEI patients' vulnerability to, 631–632

Defense mechanisms, of personality disorder patients, 633
Dementia, single-positron emission tomographic studies of, 612
Dependent personality disorder, in IEI patients, 562
Depression
  in family of IEI patients, 565
  in IEI patients, 504–505, 559, 560, 562, 563, 623, 624, 627, 628
    antidepressant therapy for, 608, 639, 640
    pancogenic challenge testing for, 532
    treatment of, 607–608
  as IEI risk factor, 501–502
  neurologic sensitization-related, 502
  as neuropsychological deficit cause, 620
  personality disorder-related, 632
  somatization associated with, 629–630
Depression spectrum disease, 565
Desensitization, as IEI treatment, 560
  psychological, 536
  systematic, 526
  through exposure, 526, 606, 607
Detoxification treatment programs, for IEI, 608
Developmental disability, as neuropsychological deficits cause, 620
Diabetes, as neuropsychological deficits cause, 620
Diagnostic evaluation, of IEI, 506, 512, 514, 539, 589, 602–606
Diagnostic Interview Schedule (DIS), 504–505, 559, 564
Diagnostic testing, of IEI patients, 604–606. *See also* Provocatvie challenge testing

Disability, IEI-related, 608, 628, 634
  government agencies' recognition of, 608
  in Gulf War veterans, 568
  iatrogenic (physician-promoted), 507
Disease, new, case definitions of, 511–512
Disease conviction, of IEI patients, 561
Displacement behavior, of IEI patients, 632
Dose-response relationship, in IEI, 499, 503, 618–619
Drugs, sensitization to. *See* Sensitization, pharmacologic
Dyspnea, IEI-related, inhalational trigger challenge testing for, 532–533

Edema, pulmonary, IEI-related, 500
Electroencephalography, quantitative, 605, 636
Electromagnetic sensitivity, of IEI patients, 630
Emotional distress, of IEI patients, 628
  dimensional assessment of, 561–562
Emotional reactions, to chemical exposure, 622
Encephalomyelitis, myalgic, IEI-associated, 630
Encephalopathy, toxic
  IEI-associated, 630
  as neuropsychological deficits cause, 620
Endotoxins, as sick building syndrome risk factor, 574
Environmental Exposure and Sensitivity Inventory (EESI), 591
Environmental tobacco smoke
  nasal resistance response to, 500, 501
  nonsmokers' *versus* smokers' olfactory thresholds for, 521
  Persian Gulf War veterans' sensitivity to, 566–567
  ventilation for control of, 579
Environment illness. *See* Idiopathic environmental intolerances (IEI)
Epilepsy, as neuropsychological deficits cause, 620
Etiological theories, of IEI, 499–506, 539–540
  behavioral theories, 499, 503–504, **521–527**
  as illness belief system, 499, 505–506. *See also* Illness belief system, of IEI patients
  as misdiagnosed psychiatric illness, 499, 504–505
  physical/toxicological mechanisms, 499–503
  immunologic theories, 499–500. *See also* Immunologic mechanisms, of IEI
  neurotoxic theories, 501–502
  nonspecific inflammation theories, 500–501
Evoked potentials, in IEI patients, 605
Executive function, neuropsychological tests for, 618
Exposure history, 602–603
Extinction, behavioral, 526
Eye irritation
  chemical exposure-related, effect of negative affectivity on, 548
  sick building syndrome-related, 574, 578, 581
  markers for, 582

Factitious disorders, in IEI patients, 634
Fatigue
  Gulf War syndrome-related, 588
  IEI-related
    IEI patients' interpretation of, 633
    pharmacological therapy for, 607–608
  sick building syndrome-related, 575
Fear, as conditioned response, 523
Fibromyalgia
  behavior therapy for, 607
  olfactory sensitivity in, 542–544
  relationship with IEI, 506, 540, 630
Food allergy
  atypical, 535
  IEI-associated, 630
  provocation challenge testing for, 653, 655
Food and Drug Administration (FDA), 612
Food aversions, conditioned, 522
Formaldehyde
  antibody assay for, 605
  exposure limits for, 576
  immunoglobulin G antibodies to, 656

Gastrointestinal tract disorders, IEI-related, 498
Generalization, in behavioral conditioning,
    520–521
  use in cognitive therapy, 526
Generalized anxiety disorder, IEI-associated, 559
  case example of, 564
  in Gulf War veterans, 567
General Medical Council of Great Britain,
    507–508
Gulf War syndrome, relationship with chemical
    sensitivity and IEI, 497, 506, **587–599**, 630
  assessment methodologies for, 591–595
  coexistent psychiatric disorders, 505
  diagnostic criteria for, 592–594
  risk factors for, 594
  symptom overlap in, 498

Headache, stereotypic stress response in, 525
Health beliefs. *See also* Illness belief system, of
    IEI patients
  effect on odor perception, 546–547
Healthcare visits, annual, by IEI patients, 508
Health risk perception, effect on odor perception,
    503–504, 545, 546–547, 557
Heavy metals exposure
  biomarkers for, 618
  as neuropsychological deficits cause, 620
Helplessness, of IEI patients, 628
Hepatic disease, as neuropsychological deficit
    cause, 620
Herbicides, neurotoxicity of, 619
Histrionic personality disorder, in IEI patients,
    562, 632, 634
Histrionic/somatizing personality style, of IEI
    patients, 563–565
Hopelessness, of IEI patients, 628
Human immunodeficiency virus infection (HIV),
    CD+ T cell deficiency associated with, 649

Humidification, as sick building syndrome cause,
    574
Huntington's disease, as neuropsychological
    deficits cause, 620
Hydrocephalus, as neuropsychological deficits
    cause, 620
Hyperosmia, 503
Hypersensitivity
  to bodily sensations, 562, 622, 633
  delayed, 649
  immediate, 649, 655
Hypertension, individual response specificity as
    risk factor for, 525
Hyperventilation
  diagnostic testing for, 560, 605
  treatment of, 607
Hypocarbia, 504
Hypochondriasis, in IEI patients, 559, 561, 562,
    565
  iatrogenic (physician-induced), 506, 560
  psychotherapy for, 641
Hypoglycemia, in IEI patients, 630
Hypothyroidism, in IEI patients, 630
Hysteria
  epidemic, 631
  historical background of, 630
  in IEI patients, 559, 561

Idea, overvalued, IEI as, 560, 633, 635, 641
Idiopathic environmental intolerances (IEI)
  case definitions of, **511–517**, 589
    in clinical studies, 511–515
    in immunologic studies, 656, 657
    in population-based studies, 515–516
  definitions of, 497, 566, 589
  diagnostic criteria for, 589
    major, 539
  as diagnostic label, 497, 515
  differentiated from objectively-defined illness,
    498
  as "fashionable" illness, 630–631
  as iatrogenic illness, 560, 567, 629, 631
  prevalence of, 498, 539
    in general population, 589
  primary gain associated with, 632, 635
  secondary gain associated with, 634
  social and political implications of, 507–508
  symptoms of, 557. *See also* specific symptoms
    commonality of, 630, 631
    as conditioned response, 523, 624
    control of, as treatment goal, 606
    IEI patients' preoccupation with, 563, 564,
      565
    onset of, 498
    patients' simulation of, 506
    relationship to chemical exposure level, 622,
      623
  treatment of, 506, 515, 606–608. *See also*
      Behavioral therapy; Cognitive-behavioral
      therapy
    symptom control goal of, 606

IEI. *See* Idiopathic environmental intolerances

Illness, psychological *versus* somatic perception of, 561

Illness belief system, of IEI patients, 499, 505–506, 560, 635
  as disability cause, 568
  expressed through membership in medical cults, 631–632
  in Gulf War veterans, 567
  iatrogenic (physician-induced), 567, 629
  Iowa Follow-up Study of, 563–565
  as projective psychological defense mechanism, 631

Immune deficiency, 649

Immunoglobulin E, as IEI marker, 657

Immunoglobulin G, as IEI marker, 654, 657

Immunoglobulin M, as IEI marker, 656

Immunologic mechanisms, of IEI, **647–665**
  conditioned immunomodulation, 521–522
  immunologic testing for, 605, 649–652
    quality control in, 652–653
    validation and evaluation of, 658–663
  studies of, 653–658
    methodologic limitations of, 656, 657, 658, 662
  theories of and evidence for, 653–658

Immunomodulation, conditioned, 521–522

Immunosciences and Specialty Laboratories, 658

Individual response specificity (IRS), 525

Inflammation, nonspecific, of respiratory mucosa, 500–501

Inhalational triggers, of IEI, use in provocative challenge testing, 532–535

Insect repellents, as Gulf War syndrome cause, 588

Intellectual ability, neuropsychological tests for, 618

International Conference on Indoor Air Quality and Climate, 580

International Society of Toxicology and Pharmacology, 507–508

Interpersonal relationships
  of IEI patients, 629
  of personality disorder patients, 633

Iowa Follow-Up Study, of persons with IEI, 563–565

Iowa Persian Gulf Study Group, 566, 594

Irritable bowel syndrome
  IEI-associated, 630
  psychotherapy for, 641

Johns Hopkins University, 658

Labels, diagnostic
  for IEI, 497, 515
  for new diseases, 511–512

Lactate, as panicogenic stimuli, 520, 529–530, 531, 536, 560

Language ability, neuropsychological tests for, 618

Language deficits, 621

Lead
  exposure limits for, 576
  neurotoxicity of, 619

Legionnaire's disease, case definition of, 515–516

Lifestyle modifications, by IEI patients
  deleterious effects of, 608
  by Gulf War veterans, 566, 567
  Iowa Follow-Up Study of, 563–565

Limbic kindling, 501–502, 535, 630

Loss-of-control, by IEI patients, 628

Malingering, by IEI patients, 634

Manganese, neurotoxicity of, 619

Manual dexterity, neuropsychological tests for, 618

Mass psychogenic illness, 550, 631

Material Safety Data Sheets, 603

Medical disorders, as neuropsychological deficits cause, 620

Medical history, of IEI patients, 602, 603–604

Medical specialties, associated with IEI etiologies, 630

Medical subculture, 505

Meditation, 636

Melancholy, 630

Memories, traumatic, 526

Memory
  IEI-related impairment of, 629
    depression-/anxiety-related, 502
  neuropsychological tests for, 618
  remote, 621

Mental model, of odor perception, 546–547

Mercury, neurotoxicity of, 619

Methyl ethyl ketone, IEI patients' olfactory sensitivity to, 540

Miller's Quick Environmental Exposure and Sensitivity Inventory (QEESI), 515

Mind-body dualism, unrealistic, in IEI patients, 628, 629

Minnesota Multiphasic Personality Inventory (MMPI), 618, 622

Moisture, as sick building syndrome risk factor, 574, 575

Mood disorders, in IEI patients, 558, 559–560, 622, 635
  neuropsychological tests for, 618
  pancogenic challenge testing of, 532
  pharmacological therapy for, 607–608

Mucocillary clearance, IEI-associated changes in, 501

Mucosal irritation. *See also* Eye irritation; Nasal irritation
  sick building syndrome-related, 574, 575
  individual susceptiblity to, 578
  low exposure-related, 581
  markers for, 582
  thermal discomfort-related, 579

Multiple chemical sensitivity. *See* Idiopathic environmental intolerances (IEI)

Multiple chemical syndrome. *See* Idiopathic environmental intolerances (IEI)

Multiple sclerosis, as neuropsychological deficits cause, 620

Narcissistic personality disorder, in IEI patients, 562, 632, 634
Nasal irritation
  chemical exposure-related, effect of attention level on, 549–550
  sick building syndrome-related, 574, 578
    markers for, 582
Nasal resistance
  in atopic patients, 574
  in IEI patients, 500–501, 540, 541
Natural killer cells, 648–649, 654
Negative affectivity
  effect on odor sensitivity, 547–549, 552
  as IEI risk factor, relationship to behavioral conditioning, 523
Neurasthenia, 506, 630, 634
Neuroimmunomodulation, 522
Neurologic disorders. *See also* Central nervous system disorders
  IEI-related, prevalence of, 498
  as neuropsychological deficits cause, 620
Neuropsychological function, of IEI patients, 502
Neuropsychological testing, in IEI, **617–625**, 629
  of affective disturbances, 622–624
  computerized, 617
  contraindication to diagnostic use of, 606
  examples of, 618
  interpretation of results in, 618–621
  sensitivity and specificity of, 621
Neurotoxic theories, of IEI, 501–502
Neutral endopeptidases, irritant exposure-related depletion of, 500
Nitrogen dioxide, exposure limits for, 576

Obsessive-compulsive disorder
  in IEI patients, 560–561, 562, 565, 622
    brain imaging studies of, 502
    as neuropsychological deficits cause, 620
Obsessive-compulsive traits, of IEI patients, 559, 634
Obsessive/paranoid personality style, of IEI patients, 562
Occupational Safety and Health Administration (OSHA), indoor air quality standard of, 581
Odor perception, as IEI trigger, 540
Odors, environmental control of, as IEI therapy, 553
Olfactory nerve, anatomic connections of, 501
Olfactory sensitivity, IEI-related, 540
  effect of attention on, 545, 549–550, 552
  effect of autonomic reactivity on, 540, 552
  comparison with fibromyalgia-related olfactory sensitivity, 542–544
  as conditioned response, 503–504, 521, 522–523, 527
  inhalational challenge trigger challenge testing of, 532–535
  effect of negative affectivity on, 547–549, 552

Olfactory sensitivity, IEI-related (*cont.*)
  nonsensory factors in, 543
  objective measures of, 543
  effect of perceived health risk on, 503–504, 545, 546–547, 552
  thresholds for, 541
  "top-down" information-processing model of, 544–552
    attention variable, 549–550, 552
    health beliefs variable, 545, 546–547, 552
    personality traits variable, 545, 547–549, 552
    socially-mediated cues variable, 545, 550–551
Operant conditioning, 526–527
Outbreak investigation paradigm, 515–516
Ozone, exposure limits for, 576

Pain, chronic
  behavior therapy for, 607
  psychotherapy for, 641
Pain threshold, of IEI patients, 633
Panic attacks
  cocaine-induced, 504
  definition of, 529
  in family of IEI patients, 565
  in IEI patients, 559, 560, 628–629
    implication for psychotherapy, 639
    panicogenic stimuli-induced, 520, 529–532, 533, 536, 560
    treatment of, 560, 607
  as neuropsychological deficits cause, 620
Panic disorder
  definition of, 529
  interoceptive conditioning in, 520
  relationship with IEI, 501–502, 504
    in Gulf War veterans, 567
  treatment model of, 638–639
  treatment of, 536
Parkinson's disease, as neuropsychological deficits cause, 620
Paroxetine, as avoidance behavior therapy, 560
Particles, exposure limits for, 576
Patient education, in IEI treatment, 553
Pavlovian conditioning, 521
  conditioned stimuli in, 520
  contextual cues in, 520
  definition of, 519–520
  extinction in, 526
  implication for IEI treatment, 525–527
  as interoceptive conditioning, 520
  in odor aversion, 523
  pharmacologic sensitization in, 524
  unconditioned stimuli in, 520
Pelvic pain, in IEI patients, 630
Permissible Exposure Levels Project, 581
Personality, components of, 632
Personality disorders. *See also* specific types of personality disorders
  exclusion from health insurance coverage, 641
  in IEI patients, 558, 559–560, 562, 568, 632–634
  prevalence of, 504–505

Personality traits
  abnormal
    of depression spectrum disorder patients, 565
    of IEI patients, 562–563
  effect on odor perception/sensitivity, 545,
    547–549
Pesticides
  as Gulf War syndrome cause, 588
  neurotoxicity of, 619
PET studies. *See* Positron emission tomography
    studies
Pharmacologic therapy. *See also* Antidepressants
  for IEI, 607–608
Phenyl ethyl alcohol, IEI patients' olfactory
    sensitivity to, 540, 541
Phobias
  in IEI patients
    aversive behavior associated with, 521
    as displaced anxiety, 628
    pancogenic challenge testing for, 532
    psychotherapy for, 641
  personality disorder-related, 632
Phobic disorder, IEI as, 504
Physical examination, of IEI patients, 602, 603
Physicians, environmental
  need for regulation of, 507
  opposition to psychotropic medication, 632
  promotion of IEI by, 629, 631
  unsubstantiated treatments provided by, 642
Physiological responses, stereotypic, to
    environmental stressors, 525
Pierce Foundation, 579
Pneumonitis, hypersensitivity, 656
Population-based studies, of IEI, 515–516
  of immunologic markers, 663
Porphyrin abnormalities
  blood enzyme assay for, 606
  IEI-associated, 630
Portland Environmental Hazards Center, 594
Positron emission tomography (PET) studies, of
    IEI, 611–612
  contraindication for diagnostic use, 615
Post-traumatic stress disorder
  behavioral conditioning basis of, 526
  exclusion from health insurance coverage, 641
  neurologic sensitization-related, 502
  as neuropsychological deficit cause, 620
  psychotherapy for, 637
  relationship with IEI, 526, 540, 639–640
    in Gulf War veterans, 566, 567
    panocogenic challenge testing for, 532
Primary gain, by IEI patients, 632, 635
Primrose oil, as IEI therapy, 563
Problem buildings. *See* Sick building syndrome
2-Propanol, IEI patients' olfactory sensitivity to,
    541, 542, 543
Provocation challenge testing, 512, 514, **529–537**
  of hypersensitivity reaction patients, 655
  with identified inhalational triggers, 532–535
    blinded inhalational challenges, 534–535
    open inhalational challenges, 532–534

Provocation challenge testing (*cont.*)
  IEI patients' rejection of results of, 633
  implication for time-dependent sensitivity, 535
  limitations of, 605
  with panicogenic substances, 529–532, 536
    intravenous sodium lactate infusion, 520,
      529–530, 531, 536, 560
    single-breath inhalation of 35 carbon
      dioxide, 529–530, 532, 536
  in patients with atypical food sensitivities, 535
  therapeutic use of, 608, 636
Provocation neutralization, 563
Psychiatric disorders
  family history of, of IEI patients, 565, 568
  in Gulf War veterans, 567, 568, 593
  IEI misdiagnosed as, 504–505
  in IEI patients
    evaluation of, 602, 604
    preexisting, 505, 558–560, 604
    prevalence of, 504–505, 557–558
    treatment of, 607
  neurologic sensitization-related, 501–502
  as neuropsychological deficits cause, 620
Psychiatric evaluation, of IEI patients, 602, 604
Psychomotor function, neuropsychological tests
    for, 618
Psychoneuroimmunology, 522
Psychosomatic illness, IEI as, 506
Psychotherapy, 636–642
  case example of, 640–641
  iatrogenic obstacles to, 631–632
  IEI patients' opposition to, 629
  insight-oriented, 635–636, 637, 638, 641
  for psychogenic IEI, **627–646**
  for sick behavior, 527
  supportive, 636
Psychotic disorders, lack of association with IEI,
    558
Psychotropic drugs. *See also* Antidepressants
  environmental physicians' opposition to, 632
  IEI patients' use of, 567, 568
Pulmonary function testing, of IEI patients, 604,
    605
Pyridostigmine, as Gulf War syndrome cause, 588

Radon, exposure limits for, 576
Randolph, Theron, 512, 630
Recall bias, in Gulf War veterans, 594
Relaxation training, 526, 536
Renal disease, as neuropsychological deficits
    cause, 620
Respirator, as hyperventilation therapy, 607
Respiratory mucosa, IEI-related nonspecific
    inflammation of, 500–501
Respiratory system disorders, IEI-related, 498
Response bias, of acetone-exposed subjects,
    546–547
Rutgers University, 658

Sarin, as Gulf War syndrome cause, 588
Schizophrenia, in IEI patients, 559, 561

Schizotypal personality disorder, in IEI patients, 562
Scripps Research Institute, 658
Secondary gain, 634
Seizures, psychogenic, 636
Selective serotonin reuptake inhibitors, 640
Self-esteem, low, of IEI patients, 628
Self-regulation therapy, for IEI, 633
Sensitization, 521
    definition of, 520
    neurologic, as IEI etiologic mechanism, 501–502
    pharmacologic, 524, 527
        to antidepressant therapy, 608
        as rationale for noncompliance with
            psychotropic medication, 632
    time-dependent, 501–502
        provocation challenge studies of, 535
Sexual abuse, childhood
    of IEI patients, 565
    as negative health perception cause, 640
Sick behaviors, reinforcement of, 527
Sick building syndrome, 497, **571–585**, 630
    engineering-related factors in, 579–580
    low-level exposure-related, 581, 582
    psychological factors in, 578–579, 582
    relationship with IEI, 498, 506
    symptoms of
        bioaerosol-related, 573, 574, 580
        documentation of, 574
        headaches, 572, 574, 575, 578
        individual susceptibility to, 578
        overlap with IEI, 498
        thermal discomfort-related, 578
        volatile organic compounds-related, 573,
            574, 575, 576–578, 580
        work stress-related, 578–579
    work-relatedness of, 573, 578–579
Sick role, of IEI patients, 628
Single-positron emission computed tomography
    (SPECT) studies, of IEI, 612, 615
    inadequate study design of, 613, 614–615
Situational response specificity (SRS), 525
Sjörgren's disease, as neuropsychological deficit
    cause, 620
Sleep disorders, as neuropsychological deficit
    cause, 620
Sleep disturbances, IEI-associated,
    pharmacological therapy for, 607–608
Social isolation, of IEI patients, 565, 628, 629,
    634
Socially-mediated cues, in chemosensory
    response, 545, 550–551
Social phobia, coexistent with IEI, pancogenic
    challenge testing for, 532
Social policy, for IEI, 507–508
Social support. *See also* Advocacy and support
    groups
    IEI patients' loss of, 608
Society of Nuclear Medicine, 612
Sodium lactate infusion, as panocgenic stimuli,
    520, 529–530, 531, 536, 560

Solvents, organic
    as cognitive deficit cause, 621
    neurotoxicity of, 619
    as panic attack cause, 504
Somatic complaints, of IEI patients, 564
Somatization
    definition of, 629
    historical background of, 630
    by IEI patients, 504, 505, 559, 561, 562,
        629–631
        Iowa Follow-Up Study of, 564, 565
        preexisting, 560
        prognosis in, 641
    personality disorder-related, 632
    psychotherapy guidelines for, 635
Somatoform disorders
    exclusion from health insurance coverage, 641
    in IEI patients, 558, 559–560, 568
        pancogenic challenge testing for, 532
    as neuropsychological deficit cause, 620
    somatization associated with, 629–630
    somatization diagnosed as, 629
    treatment resistance in, 640
SPECT studies. *See* Single positron emission
    computed tomography (SPECT) studies
Stimuli. *See also* Behavioral conditioning;
    Pavlovian conditioning
    new, generalization response to, 520–521
    noxious, sensitization response to, 520
Stress
    effect on olfactory sensitivity, 503
    personality disorder patients' response to, 633
    effect on pharmacologic conditioning, 524
    work-related, physical symptoms of, 578–579
Stress management, by IEI patients, 608, 636, 639
Stroke, brain imaging-assisted diagnosis of, 612
Structured Interview for DSM-II-R Personality
    Disorders, 504–505
Subculture, medical, 505
Sublingual neutralization, 608
Substance abuse. *See also* Alcohol
    abuse/alcoholism
    by family of IEI patients, 565
    lack of association wit IEI, 558, 560
Substance P, nasal effects of, 500, 501
Suggestibility threshold, of IEI patients, 633
Suicide attempts, 565
Sulfur dioxide, exposure limits for, 576
Support and advocacy groups, 551, 563, 564, 629,
    631–632, 633, 634
Symptom Checklist-90-revised (SCL-90-R), 618
Symptom diary, 603
Systemic lupus erythematosus, as
    neuropsychological deficits cause, 620

Taste aversion, conditioned, 522
T cells. *See also* specific types of CD T cells
    in IEI, 653, 654, 657
    immune function of, 648
20th-century disease. *See* Idiopathic
    environmental intolerances (IEI)

Thermal discomfort, in buildings, 578, 579–580
Throat symptoms, IEI-related, inhalational trigger challenge testing for, 532–534
Thyroid dysfunction, as neuropsychological deficits cause, 620
Toluene diisocyanate, immunoglobulin G antibodies to, 656
Total allergy syndrome. *See* Idiopathic environmental intolerances (IEI)
Transactions of the American Society for Ventilating Engineers, 579

Unemployment
  of Gulf War veterans, 568
  of IEI patients, 608
U. S. Department of Defense, Comprehensive Clinical Evaluation Program, 588
U. S. Department of Veterans Affairs, Gulf War Registry of, 588, 589, 590, 591, 592, 595
Universal allergy. *See* Idiopathic environmental intolerances (IEI)
University of Washington, 658
Unmasking, 589
Upper respiratory tract, IEI-associated nonspecific inflammation of, 500–501

Ventilation
  for environmental tobacco smoke control, 579
Ventilation, as sick building syndrome cause, 574, 579, 580
Verbal memory, neuropsychological tests for, 618
Victimization, of IEI patients, 628, 629
Viral infections, as neuropsychological deficits cause, 620
Visuoconstruction/visuoperception, neuropsychological tests for, 618
Volatile organic compounds (VOCs)
  as sick building syndrome cause, 573, 574, 575, 576–578, 580
  structure-activity relationship of, 575

Withdrawal symptoms, as neuropsychological deficits cause, 620
Workers' compensation, for IEI, 507, 634
Workplace, chemical exposure control in, 607
World Health Organization (WHO)
  International Programme on Chemical Safety of, 511
  position statement on IEI, 507–508

"Yeast connection," of IEI, 630